Standard Operational Procedures in Reproductive Medicine

Laboratory and Clinical Practice

REPRODUCTIVE MEDICINE AND ASSISTED REPRODUCTIVE TECHNIQUES SERIES

David Gardner
University of Melbourne, Australia

Zeev Shoham
Kaplan Hospital, Rehovot, Israel

Kay Elder, Jacques Cohen
Human Preimplantation Embryo Selection, ISBN: 9780415399739

John D Aplin, Asgerally T Fazleabas, Stanley R Glasser, Linda C Giudice
The Endometrium, Second Edition, ISBN: 9780415385831

Nick Macklon, Ian Greer, Eric Steegers
Textbook of Periconceptional Medicine, ISBN: 9780415458924

Andrea Borini, Giovanni Coticchio
Preservation of Human Oocytes, ISBN: 9780415476799

Steven R Bayer, Michael M Alper, Alan S Penzias
The Boston IVF Handbook of Infertility, Third Edition, ISBN: 9781841848105

Ben Cohlen, Willem Ombelet
Intra-Uterine Insemination: Evidence Based Guidelines for Daily Practice,
ISBN: 9781841849881

Adam H. Balen
Infertility in Practice, Fourth Edition, ISBN: 9781841848495

Nick Macklon
IVF in the Medically Complicated Patient, Second Edition:
A Guide to Management, ISBN: 9781482206692

Michael Tucker, Juergen Liebermann
Vitrification in Assisted Reproduction, ISBN: 9780415408820

Ben J Cohlen, Evert J P van Santbrink, Joop S E Laven
Ovulation Induction: Evidence Based Guidelines for Daily Practice,
ISBN: 9781498704076

Botros Rizk, Markus Montag
Standard Operational Procedures in Reproductive Medicine:
Laboratory and Clinical Practice,
ISBN: 9781498719216

Standard Operational Procedures in Reproductive Medicine

Laboratory and Clinical Practice

Edited by

Botros Rizk, MD, FRCOG, FRCS, HCLD, FACOG, FACS
Professor and Head of Reproductive Endocrinology and Infertility
Medical and Scientific Director of In Vitro Fertilization and Assisted Reproduction
University of South Alabama
Mobile, Alabama, USA

Distinguished Adjunct Professor of Reproductive Endocrinology and Infertility
Obstetrics and Gynecology
King Abdulaziz University
Jeddah, Kingdom of Saudi Arabia

Distinguished Adjunct Scientific Director
IVF Michigan
Rochester Hills, Michigan, USA

Markus Montag, PhD
Professor and CEO
ilabcomm GmbH
Sankt Augustin, NRW, Germany

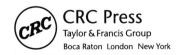

CRC Press
Taylor & Francis Group
Boca Raton London New York

CRC Press is an imprint of the
Taylor & Francis Group, an **informa** business

CRC Press
Taylor & Francis Group
6000 Broken Sound Parkway NW, Suite 300
Boca Raton, FL 33487-2742

© 2017 by Taylor & Francis Group, LLC
CRC Press is an imprint of Taylor & Francis Group, an Informa business

No claim to original U.S. Government works

Printed on acid-free paper

International Standard Book Number-13: 978-1-4987-1921-6 (Paperback)

Visit the Taylor & Francis Web site at
http://www.taylorandfrancis.com

and the CRC Press Web site at
http://www.crcpress.com

To my father, Mitry Botros Rizk, 1916–2003, a great and most caring man

who inspired me every day of my life and lived to do that.

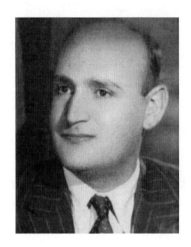

Contents

Section II   Clinical Procedures

About the Editors

Botros Rizk is Professor and Head of Reproductive Endocrinology and Infertility and Medical and Scientific Director of In Vitro Fertilization and Assisted Reproduction at the University of South Alabama. Dr. Rizk is distinguished Adjunct Professor of Reproductive Endocrinology and Infertility Obstetrics and Gynecology in King Abdulaziz University, Jeddah, Kingdom of Saudi Arabia. Dr. Rizk is distinguished Adjunct Scientific Director of IVF at Michigan Rochester Hills. He is also President elect of the Middle East Fertility Society.

Mentored by Nobel Laureate Professor Robert Edwards, recipient of the Nobel Prize in Medicine for achieving the first successful in vitro fertilization in the world, Dr. Rizk started his career in Reproductive Medicine in London and Cambridge, where most of the current scientific developments and medical protocols were invented. He joined the prestigious University of Cambridge for three years from 1990 to 1993. Dr. Rizk is board certified by the American Board of Obstetrics and Gynecology and the Royal College of Physicians and Surgeons of Canada and the Royal College of Obstetricians and Gynaecologist in England, as well as the American Board of Bioanalysts in Embryology and Andrology.

Dr. Rizk's clinical and research interests have focused on ovarian stimulation, including the development of the long agonist protocol inspired by his colleagues Professors Howard Jacobs and Seang Lin Tan and Charles Kingsland in London. He is internationally considered a leading authority on ovarian hyperstimulation syndrome and made original contributions to the pathophysiology and prevention of the syndrome. Dr. Rizk authored a book solely dedicated to ovarian hyperstimulation syndrome that is considered the standard reference for OHSS. Dr. Rizk is an authority on endometriosis, its novel medical management and robotic surgery.

Professor Rizk has edited and authored 20 medical textbooks and more than 400 manuscripts embracing different aspects of infertility and assisted reproduction, as well as ultrasonography and robotic surgery. Dr. Rizk is one of the early members of the European Society for Human Reproduction and a founding member of the Middle East Fertility Society. He chaired for several years many ASRM postgraduate courses teaching ART, ovarian stimulation and ultrasonography.

Markus Montag started his career at the German Cancer Research Centre in developmental biology. He continued as post-doc in the team of Prof S.C. Ng, the father of the first SUZI baby at the National University Hospital Singapore. In 1993 he started as laboratory director in IVF, first in a private IVF unit, then at the University of Bonn from 1995 to 2011, and finally at the University of Heidelberg until 2013. Since 2013 he has served as CEO of his consultancy company called ilabcomm.

He has published more than 200 peer-reviewed articles, 20 book chapters and started editing his own books. He is involved worldwide in counselling IVF centers, lecturing and educating young people.

He was involved in the introduction of laser technology in the IVF laboratory, the establishment of the ESHRE trial on polar body biopsy and array CGH for PGS and he is a co-founder of the German network for fertility protection for women (FertiPROTEKT). His major topics of interest are the identification of the potential of embryos, time-lapse technology and ovarian tissue banking.

List of Contributors

Ahmed Abdelaziz
Department of Obstetrics and Gynecology
Hurley Medical Center
Michigan State University College of Human Medicine
Flint, Michigan

Mostafa Abuzeid
Reproductive Endocrinology and Infertility
Hurley Medical Center
Michigan State University College of Human Medicine
Flint, Michigan
IVF Michigan Rochester Hills & Flint
PC, Rochester Hills, Michigan

Omar Abuzeid
Department of Obstetrics and Gynecology
Hurley Medical Center
Michigan State University College of Human Medicine
Flint, Michigan

Ashok Agarwal
Andrology Laboratory
Cleveland Clinic
Cleveland, Ohio

Gautam N. Allahbadia
Rotunda—The Center For Human Reproduction
Mumbai, India
Aster IVF & Women Clinic
Dubai, UAE

Oscar D. Almeida, Jr.
Department of Obstetrics and Gynecology
University of South Alabama Children and Women's
    Hospital
Mobile, Alabama

Daniel Antonious
Department of Obstetrics and Gynecology
University of South Alabama
Mobile, Alabama

Baris Ata
Department of Obstetrics and Gynecology
Koç University School of Medicine
Istanbul, Turkey

Shawky Z.A. Badawy
Department of Obstetrics and Gynecology
Department of Clinical Pathology
Reproductive Endocrinology and Infertility
SUNY Upstate Medical University
Syracuse, New York

Basak Balaban
Assisted Reproduction Unit
VKF American Hospital
Istanbul, Turkey

Arsany Bassily
Department of Obstetrics and Gynecology
University of South Alabama
Mobile, Alabama

Vera Baukloh
IVF Laboratory
Fertility Center Hamburg
Hamburg, Germany

Barry Behr
Division of Reproductive Endocrinology and Infertility
Department of Obstetrics and Gynecology
Stanford University Medical Center
Stanford, California

Alan Bolnick
Division of Reproductive Endocrinology and Infertility,
    Department of OB/GYN
Wayne State University School of Medicine
Detroit, Michigan

Linda D. Bradley
Obstetrics & Gynecology and Women's Health Institute
Cleveland Clinic
Cleveland, Ohio

Brian Brocato
Department of Obstetrics and Gynecology
Division of Maternal Fetal Medicine
University of South Alabama
Mobile, Alabama

Mariabeatrice Dal Canto
Biogenesi Reproductive Medicine Centre
Istituti Clinici Zucchi
Monza, Italy

Robert F. Casper
Department of Obstetrics and Gynecology
University of Toronto
and
Lunenfeld-Tanenbaum Research Institute
and
TRIO Fertility, Toronto
and
Insception-Lifebank Cord Blood Bank
Toronto, Canada

Jana Claeys
Department of Obstetrics and Gynecology
University Hospital Ghent
Ghent, Belgium

Ana Cobo
IVI Valencia
Cryobiology Unit-IVF laboratory
Valencia, Spain

Aila Coello
IVI Valencia
Cryobiology Unit-IVF laboratory
Valencia, Spain

Giovanni Coticchio
Biogenesi Reproductive Medicine Centre
Istituti Clinici Zucchi
Monza, Italy

Michael H. Dahan
OriginElle Fertility Clinic & Women Health Centre
Montreal, Canada
Department of Obstetrics and Gynecology McGill
    University
Montreal, Canada

Christian De Geyter
Clinic of Gynecological Endocrinology and Reproductive
    Medicine
University Hospital of Basel
Basel, Switzerland

Maria De Geyter
Clinic of Gynecological Endocrinology and Reproductive
    Medicine
University Hospital of Basel
Basel, Switzerland

Michael Dooley
The Poundbury Clinic
Dorchester, United Kingdom
The Poundbury Suite
King Edward VII Hospital
London, United Kingdom

Thomas Ebner
Department of Gynecology, Obstetrics and Gynecological
    Endocrinology
Kepler University
Linz, Austria

Joshua Ekladios
Department of Obstetrics and Gynecology
University of South Alabama
Mobile, Alabama

Islam Fahmi
Department of Obstetrics and Gynecology
Hurley Medical Center
Michigan State University College of Human Medicine
Flint, Michigan

Thomas Freour
Service de médecine de la reproduction
CHU de Nantes
and
INSERM UMR1064
and
Faculté de médecine
Université de Nantes
Nantes, France

Goral N. Gandhi
Rotunda—The Center For Human Reproduction
Mumbai, India

Juan Antonio García-Velasco
IVI Madrid
Rey Juan Carlos University
Madrid, Spain

Jan Gerris
Division of Reproductive Medicine and Women's Clinic
University Hospital Ghent
Ghent, Belgium

Martin Greuner
IVF-SAAR Saarbrücken-Kaiserslautern
Saarbrücken, Germany

Thorir Hardarson
IVF Sweden
Stockholm, Sweden

Cristina Hickman
Boston Place Clinic
The Fertility Partnership
London, United Kingdom

Candice P. Holliday
Department of Obstetrics and Gynecology
University of South Alabama
Mobile, Alabama

Julius Hreinsson
IVF Sweden
Stockholm, Sweden

Carin Huyser
Reproductive Biology Laboratory
Reproductive and Endocrine Unit
Department of Obstetrics and Gynaecology
University of Pretoria
Steve Biko Academic Hospital
Pretoria, South Africa

Graciela Kohls Ilgner
IVI Madrid
Madrid, Spain

Lars Johansson
Centre of Reproduction
Women's Clinic, Academic Hospital
Uppsala, Sweden

Salem Joseph
IVF Michigan Rochester Hills and Flint
Flint, Michigan

Semra Kahraman
Istanbul Memorial Hospital
ART and Reproductive Genetics Center
Istanbul, Turkey

Rabea Youcef Khoudja
OriginElle Fertility Clinic & Women Health Centre
Montreal, Canada

Kiranpreet Khurana
Department of Urology
Cleveland Clinic
Cleveland, Ohio

Borut Kovačič
Reproductive Medicine & Gynecologic Endocrinology
University Medical Centre Maribor
Maribor, Slovenia

Alex Lagunov
CCRM Toronto/Hannam Fertility Center
Toronto, Canada

David F. Lewis
Department of Obstetrics and Gynecology
LSU Health
Shreveport, Louisiana

Spiros A. Liatsikos
Centre for Reproduction and Advanced Technology
    "CREATE Fertility"
London, United Kingdom

Jana Liebenthron
Gynecological Endocrinology and Reproductive Medicine
University of Bonn
Bonn, Germany

Megan Lively
Department of Obstetrics and Gynecology
University of South Alabama
Mobile, Alabama

Hashem Lotfy
Department of Obstetrics and Gynecology
University of South Alabama
Mobile, Alabama
and
Department of Obstetrics and Gynecology
Tanta University
Tanta, Egypt

Lauren Mann
Department of Obstetrics and Gynecology
University of South Alabama
Mobile, Alabama

Marius Meintjes
Frisco Institute for Reproductive Medicine
Frisco, Texas

Magued Adel Mikhail
Assisted Conception Unit
Guy's and Saint Thomas Hospital
London, United Kingdom
and
Department of Obstetrics and Gynecology
University of South Alabama
Mobile, Alabama

Andrew Mok
OriginElle Fertility Clinic & Women Health Centre
and
Department of Obstetrics and Gynecology
McGill University
Montreal, Canada

Markus Montag
ilabcomm GmbH
Sankt Augustin, Germany

Dean E. Morbeck
Fertility Associates
Auckland, New Zealand

David Mortimer
Oozoa Biomedical Inc
Vancouver, Canada

Sharon T. Mortimer
Oozoa Biomedical Inc
Vancouver, Canada

Geeta Nargund
Centre for Reproduction and Advanced Technology
    "CREATE Fertility"
London, United Kingdom

Verena Nordhoff
Centre of Reproductive Medicine and Andrology
Department of Clinical and Operative Andrology
University Hospital of Münster
Münster, Germany

Bolonduro Oluwamuyiwa
Department of OB/GYN
Mayo Clinic Health System
Austin Campus, Minnesota
Austin, Minnesota

Willem Ombelet
Department of Obstetrics and Gynaecology
Ziekenhuizen Oost-Limburg
and
Genk Institute for Fertilitity Technologies
and
Faculty of Medicine and Life Sciences
Hasselt University
Diepenbeek, Belgium

Rubin Raju
Department of Obstetrics and Gynecology
Mayo School of Medicine
Rochester, Minnesota
Mayo Clinic Health Systems
Red Wing, Minnesota

Botros Rizk
Department of Obstetrics and Gynecology
University of South Alabama
Mobile, Alabama
and
King Abdulaziz University
Jeddah, Kingdom of Saudi Arabia
and
OriginElle USA
Dallas, Texas
and
Middle East Fertility Society
Cairo, Egypt

Edmund Sabanegh, Jr.
Department of Urology
Cleveland Clinic
Cleveland, Ohio

Denny Sakkas
Boston IVF
Waltham, Massachusetts

Wael Salem
Reproductive Endocrinology and Infertility
UCSF Center for Reproductive Health
San Francisco, California

Hassan N. Sallam
Department of Obstetrics and Gynaecology
University of Alexandria and Alexandria Fertility and IVF
    Center
Alexandria, Egypt

Nooman H. Sallam
Department of Obstetrics and Gynaecology
University of Alexandria and Alexandria Fertility and IVF
    Center
Alexandria, Egypt

Rahima Sanya
Department of Obstetrics and Gynecology
Hurley Medical Center
Michigan State University College of Human Medicine
Flint, Michigan

Ippokratis Sarris
Centre for Reproduction and Advanced Technology
    "CREATE Fertility"
London, United Kingdom

James M. Shwayder
Department of Obstetrics and Gynecology
University of Mississippi Medical Center
Jackson, Mississippi

Jason E. Swain
CCRM IVF Network
Lone Tree, Colorado

Nayana Talukdar
Division of Reproductive Sciences
University of Toronto, Lunenfeld-Tanenbaum Research
    Institute, Mount Sinai Hospital
and
TCART Fertility Partners
Toronto, Canada

Justin Tan
Department of Obstetrics and Gynecology
University of British Colombia
Vancouver, Canada

Seang Lin Tan
OriginElle Fertility Clinic & Women Health Centre
and
Department of Obstetrics and Gynecology
McGill University
Montreal, Canada

Bettina Toth
Department of Gynecological Endocrinology and
    Reproductive Medicine
Medical University of Innsbruck
Innsbruck, Austria

Rola Turki
Department of Obstetrics and Gynecology
King Abdulaziz University
Jeddah, Saudi Arabia
and
Department of Obstetrics and Gynecology
University of South Alabama
Mobile, Alabama

Etienne Van den Abbeel
Department of Reproductive Medicine
University Hospital Gent
Gent, Belgium

Hakan Yelke
Istanbul Memorial Hospital
ART and Reproductive Genetics Center
Istanbul, Turkey

Osama A.H. Abu Zinadah
Department of Biological Sciences
King Abdulaziz University
Jeddah, Saudi Arabia

Section I

Laboratory Procedures

1

The Documentation System

Markus Montag and Lars Johansson

Standard operational procedures (SOPs) are one part of the whole documentation system in the reproductive laboratory.

Purpose of a Documentation System

- Tracking patient therapy
- Tracking all processes in relation to methods and organization within a laboratory
- Tracking all involved personnel and material
- Enabling internal and external communication and QC
- Evaluating and optimizing processes and techniques

Formal Aspects of Documentation

- Documents have to be continuously updated and linked to corresponding documents and must be ordered to reflect the documentation/treatment chain.
- Documents must all follow the same layout.
- Actual documents ought to be available both as hard copy in a folder and as an on-screen version.
- Outdated documents must be archived in chronological order.

Document Structure

- Document name: name under which the document is saved/additional elements to characterize status (e.g., "archived" for a document that is no longer in use or has been updated)
- Title of the document: related to the purpose
- Document number: unique number for easy recovery
- Purpose of the document: what the document is dealing with
- Date of release: date from which the document is implemented/valid
- Version: starting with version 1; higher numbers indicate updated versions/revisions
- Number of pages: total number as well as an indication of the present page

SOPs and Related Documents

- Describe a procedure or process and how it has to be performed by everyone.
- Procedures can be of laboratory or technical (equipment) nature.
- Procedures include detailed aspects that are important for running a smooth lab operation, for example:
  - How to order products.
  - How to release new products for routine clinical use.
  - How to retrieve samples (e.g., testicular tissue) from external sources.
  - How to ship materials (e.g., cryopreserved samples).
  - How to deal with emergency situations (e.g., dish flipped on the floor/power failure/gas supply failure/alarm situation/...).
- Procedures have to be trained and competency tests performed annually, thus a document/SOP on training, education and release of personnel has to be in place, as well as a document that documents the training process.
- SOPs that describe how to perform a procedure (e.g., ICSI) have to name the accompanying (patient-related) documents in which the procedure must be documented.
- SOPs allow checks for procedure compliance and are the base for audits.

Figure 1.1. shows the sample layout for a SOP that applies to a laboratory procedure (like ICSI).

Clinic Emblem IVF-Lab- **Clinic Name—1.001 SOP layout**

Title / Name: Example of a SOP	
SOP: 1.001_SOP layout	Version: 1

Purpose or topic of the document

Materials and Devices used

Preparation on the day before

Preparation on the same day

Detailed description of the procedure

Special Note

Related documents (preferably using a link)

Documentation requirements

	Name	Date (dd/mm/yyyy)	Signature
Prepared By			
Original Date			
Revision Dates			
Effective dates			
Review Date			
Approvals			
Lab Director			
Medical Director			

FIGURE 1.1 Sample SOP Layout

2

Culture Media Techniques

Lars Johansson

Culture in Single-Step Media Versus Sequential Media

- The culture from 2PN (zygote) stage to blastocyst on day 5/6 can either be performed in single-step or sequential culture media.
  - The single-step culture media decrease the environmental stress, the nutrition (paracrine and autocrine factors) is not removed, and it demands less work, is less costly and seems to generate more blastocysts.
  - Sequential media culture takes into consideration the changes in metabolism and environment that the embryos encounter during their development.
- Embryos are either cultured individually or in groups and preferably in droplets. Individual culture allows successively evaluating embryo development and quality to ease the selection of the best embryo(s) for transfer.
  - Group culture allows the exchange of nutrients between the embryos, whereby high concentrations of autocrine and paracrine embryo-trophic and detoxifying factors surround the embryos.
  - A high density of embryos generates higher concentrations of embryo-trophic factors, but also a potential enrichment of detrimental waste products that could be dependent on media product and culture technique.
  - Group culture cannot rectify for poor design of clinic, air quality, selection of equipment and disposables and bad stimulation, egg retrieval and culture techniques.

Equipment

- Laminar flow (LAF) bench, class II cabinet or IVF chamber with a built in stereo microscope, a calibrated, heated surface and light source and optionally a temperature-controlled humidified media-specific mix of gas (adjusted to the type of media used and altitude level of the clinic).
- Incubators with small inner doors set at an appropriate percentage of CO_2 and low oxygen (O_2).
- Bench-top mini-incubator; supported by a pre-mixed gas ($CO_2/O_2/N_2$) or gas from a gas-mixer.
- Time-lapse incubators for continuous evaluation and culture of embryos at low oxygen.
- Labelling machine: for creation of patient-specific identification labels for the dishes.
- Pipette aid: For transfer of pre-incubated oil or large volumes of culture media.
- Multidispenser pipettes.
- General autoclave pipettes.

Disposables

All disposables should be sterile, embryo-tested, VOC-free, non-pyrogenic and gamma-sterilized.

- Center-well dishes (60 mm)—for insemination or culture
- Culture dishes (35 mm, 40 mm, 60 mm, four-five-well, micro-droplet or time-lapse dish)
- Filter tips: irradiated, sterile filter tips free of pyrogens, RNases and DNases
- Pipette tips: CombiTips, PCR Clean and single wrapped (1–50 mL sizes), for repeater pipettes
- Serological pipettes: 5 and 10 mL or use of sterile plastic Pasteur pipettes
- Gloves: embryo-tested powder-free sterile gloves without chemical additives, accelerants or emulsifiers
- Media and embryo handling pipettes: for single use; sterile with a filter
- Detergent: cleaning solution for laboratory surfaces, equipment and in between patients
- Lint-free wipes for cleaning
- Aqua ad injectionem for cleaning purposes and incubators

- Culture media products of your choice: sequential or single-step medium
- Patient-specific identification and culture media documentation (protocols)

General Considerations While Working with Culture Media

- Culture media products must be stored and handled properly and used within given expiry dates and days after opening.
- Oocytes and embryos must be kept at optimal culture conditions (superior gas quality, pH, humidity, low oxygen tension, temperature, low number of incubator door openings).
- Avoid exposure of culture media and embryos to environmental embryo-toxic pollutants.
- For each patient, pre-ventilated dishes are prepared in a serviced and calibrated LAF bench or class II cabinet using a regimen that warrants low VOC contamination.
- Label dishes, both lid and bottom, with the couple's specific barcode identifier, or chip and number the droplets for easy identification.
- Avoid using label pens since toxins from the paint fume off inside the incubator.
- Keep the heated surface area and the light source off while preparing dishes!
- Turn on the ventilation of the LAF bench or class II cabinet long before the surface area is cleaned so that dirt or particles, from the HEPA filter, are prevented from contaminating the surface area or the dishes.
- Use a low fan speed to reduce evaporation rates of the media during the preparation of the dishes.
- Clean the surface area with water for injection and lint-free clean-room wipes only!
- Put on embryo-tested sterile gloves and work aseptically.
- Place the pre-ventilated culture dishes, pipettes, repeater pipettes, CombiTips and filter tips on the surface of the LAF bench or the class II cabinet.
- Clean the outer parts of all pipettes with wipes moist with water for injection if necessary.
- Adjust the number of dishes according to the number of expected 2PN and culture techniques.
- Pre-rinse all pipettes or syringes, with their designated media, just before use to avoid drying in of media, potential crystal formation and increase in osmolality.
- Take out your choice of culture media, one at a time, from the refrigerator and place the media on the cold and clean surface of the LAF bench or in the bottom part of a large Petri dish.

- Pre-incubated liquid paraffin oil (PLPO) is taken out from the incubator and placed in the bottom part of a large sterile Petri dish.
- Attach a suitable CombiTip to the repeater pipette or use standard pipettes.
- Aspirate medium and pre-rinse the pipette-tip with the selected culture media, refill the pipette.
- Prepare one dish at a time, especially if low-volume media droplets are prepared.
- Cover media droplets or media immediately with oil before preparing another dish.
- **Note:** When using dry incubation conditions, oil is a must.
- All dishes must be pre-incubated overnight for at least 8 hours to ensure correct pH of the media.
- The same procedure is used for preparing dishes for culture with a single-step or sequential media.

Time Course for Preparation of Dishes

- In the afternoon of the day of egg collection: Prepare and pre-incubate the culture dishes overnight for the zygotes.
- Culture dishes for sequential cultures are prepared and pre-incubated overnight.
- **Note:** Some clinics routinely exchange cleavage-stage medium for blastocyst medium on day 3, others on day 2 in the early afternoon.
- Embryo transfer dish: Always prepare in the afternoon on the day before transfer.

How to Prepare Different Types of Dishes Independent of Culture Strategy

- Culture in center-well dishes.
  - Fill the outer ring with ca 1.5 mL and the inner well with 600–1800 µL of medium.
  - Cover the inner center-well with a thin layer of PLPO.
  - Some clinics only use media droplets (20–50 µL) in the inner center-well, which are covered with a thin film of PLPO with a sterile serological pipette or Pasteur pipette.
- Culture in Petri dishes (35–60 mm).
  - Select a flat-bottom dish with a good contact to the heated surface of the incubators for quicker recovery of the culture conditions.
  - **Note:** Be aware of the edge effect (optimal interference and temperature drops) and only use flat-bottom dishes with clear visibility!
  - Prepare a suitable number of culture dishes adjusted to your culture routines and label accordingly.
- Culture in four- to five-well dishes.

- Fill 500–1000 μL in each straight-wall well of the dish. Some five-well dishes have a sloped wall, which makes it also possible to use for smaller droplets.
- Cover the droplets with oil with a sterile serological or Pasteur pipette.
- Culture in specially designed dishes (GPS dishes/micro-droplet dishes/time-lapse dishes).
  - Prepare specially designed dishes according to the recommendations by the manufacturer.
  - Air bubbles may present a problem, therefore take care to remove them the next day, prior to use of the dish.

BIBLIOGRAPHY

Alpha Scientists in Reproductive Medicine and ESHRE Special Interest Group Embryology. 2011. "Istanbul Consensus Workshop on Embryo Assessment: Proceedings of an Expert Meeting." *Reproductive Biomedicine Online* 22: 632–46.

Montag, M., ed. *A Practical Guide to Selecting Gametes and Embryos*. Taylor & Francis Group, CRC Press, 2014.

Quinn, P., ed. *Culture Media, Solutions and Systems in Human ART*. Cambridge University Press, 2014.

Smith, G.D., J.E. Swain, and T.B. Pool, eds. *Embryo Culture: Methods and Protocols*. Humana Press, Springer Science + Business Media, 2012.

3

IVF Incubator Handling

Jason E. Swain and Alex Lagunov

Setup

Required Equipment

- Incubator (low-oxygen incubators should be standard for all IVF procedures)
- 1/4″ ID Tygon tubing
- Tubing fasteners or zip-ties
- Inline VOC gas filter
- Medical grade gases (CO_2, nitrogen or premixed cylinders)
- Gas regulators

Setting Up Incubator

- Incubator should be cleaned (see "Cleaning the incubator").
- Attach regulators to gas cylinders and set appropriate gas pressure according to incubator requirements before connecting to the incubator.
- Place incubator in a low-traffic area within the lab. Incubator should be raised off the floor, preferably on a counter top or on a raised cart/stand.
- Ensure that the incubator is not directly below any air vents.
- Attach appropriate extensions of Tygon tubing and secure to the gas regulator, whether piped through from a manifold or directly connected to the tank.
- Install inline gas filtration in the existing Tygon tubing and secure.
- Attach and secure Tygon tubing to the appropriate inlet of the incubator (CO_2, N_2 or mixed).
- Turn on incubator, preferably plugged into an outlet connected to a back-up power generator. Do not turn on the gas supply yet.
- Adjust temperature to "burn in" the incubator (commonly $\geq 50°C$) 7–14 days.
- After "burn in", set temperature to 37°C and validate temperature using an NBS/NIST calibrated independent thermometer.

- Ensure gas pressure is set to incubator requirements. Failure to do so can damage the incubator. This can be done at the gas supply itself, or more commonly with a step-down regulator at the gas outlet within the lab.
- Once gas outlet pressure is confirmed, turn on gas supply and set appropriate gas concentrations on the incubator to achieve the desired media pH.
- Confirm gas measurement (see "Gas measurements") and pH (see "pH measurements").
- Perform an appropriate bioassay prior to use with human samples (a 1-cell MEA is preferred, with >70% blastocyst formation).

Gas Measurements

Required Equipment

- Gas analyzer (automatic gas analyzers are recommended over manual Fyrite analyzers)
- Tubing for automatic gas analyzer connection
- 0.2 micron filter or moisture trap (required for humidified incubators using an automatic gas analyzer)
- Daily incubator QC paperwork

Preparation on the Day of Use

- Gas reading must be performed first thing in the morning prior to incubator opening.
- Ensure gas analyzer or Fyrite are up to date with calibrations or solution replacement.
- Ensure analyzers are zeroed prior to use.

Measuring Gas

- Must be performed for every incubator, every morning of use.

- Attach sample tube to the incubator gas sampling port.
- Follow instructions supplied by the specific gas analyzer.
  - Manually pump Fyrite for both oxygen and CO_2 and invert the correct number of times. Read the top of the meniscus.
  - Turn on the fan pump for automated gas analyzers. Let the analyzer run for the same amount of time for each incubator to stabilize gas readings (approximately 3 min).
- Record gas readings (CO_2 and oxygen) for each incubator on the incubator daily log. If gas readings are out of range, re-sample. If still out of range, take corrective action.
  - Corrective actions may include moving cells to another incubator, verifying gas sensor function, replacing gas sensor, or adjusting gas concentration.

pH Measurements

Required Equipment

- pH meter or blood gas analyzer (pH meter must have a functioning probe. Glass double junction KCl filled is recommended. Probe should be replaced annually)
- Test tubes/culture dishes
- pH standards for calibration (pH meter)
- Warming block (pH meter)
- Incubator QC paperwork
- Culture media with protein
- 1 cc syringe (blood gas analyzer)

Preparation the Day Before

- Place culture media with protein added into each incubator in a loosely capped test tube or other appropriate dish. Oil must be used if testing a non-humidifed incubator.

Preparation on the Day

- If using a pH meter:
  - Aliquot pH standards 7 and 10 into test tubes and warm to 37°C the day of use.
  - Calibrate pH meter according to instrument instruction. Slope must be in acceptable range (98–102).
  - Check calibration by re-measuring pH 7 standard. Value should be 6.98–7.02. If out of range, recalibrate.
- If using blood gas analyzer:

- Ensure test cards or cartridges are available and analyzer is powered on and functioning.

Measuring pH

- If using a pH meter:
  - Media tube should be quickly removed from one incubator, capped and quickly taken to the pH meter.
  - Place probe into the test tube and record pH.
- Repeat for all other incubators.
- If using a blood gas analyzer:
  - Insert a new cartridge into the analyzer, allow it to calibrate.
  - Once calibration is complete, quickly prepare to load the sample.
  - Remove media tube or dish from incubator.
  - Draw up media in the 1 cc syringe (approximately 0.3 mL).
  - Remove needle and inject the appropriate amount of media into the cartridge inserted in the blood gas analyzer to obtain the pH reading.
- If pH is out of the acceptable range, examine gas readings. Remake media and retest pH later in the day if possible. If still out of range, take corrective action, which may entail adjusting incubator CO_2 levels (raise CO_2 to lower pH and lower CO_2 to raise pH). Relocate cells until problem has been resolved and pH is back into normal range (normal range varies and is media and lab dependent).

Note: pH should be measured at regular intervals. While daily or weekly pH measurement may be useful, pH should be measured at a minimum when using a new lot of culture media and after incubator shutdown/cleaning.

Cleaning Laboratory Incubators

Required Equipment

- Cleaning/disinfecting agent (hydrogen peroxide or other low-VOC agent; ethanol is not recommended)
- Spray bottle or bucket
- Sterile surgical towel or gauze pads
- Autoclave system (*optional*)
- Autoclave tape (*optional*)
- Autoclave wrap (*optional*)
- Sterile distilled water
- Gloves (non-powder)
- Documentation chart/QC paperwork

Preparation on the Day

- Fill spray bottle or bucket with appropriate cleaning agent.

- Set out surgical towel or gauze.
- Follow manufacturer's instructions regarding electrical shutdown of unit. This is most important in incubators with internal fans. Additionally, shutdown of gas supply can be performed to conserve resources.

Cleaning the Incubator

Note: Cleaning should be performed on a regular basis. Water pans, if present, should be emptied and replaced with clean water every 2–4 weeks. At a minimum, a thorough cleaning should be performed annually, including a complete breakdown of all internal pieces. A more regular, quarterly or biannual cleaning is recommended. Quarterly/biannual cleanings do not necessarily require a complete incubator disassembly and a thorough surface/interior wipe may be sufficient. Which incubators are cleaned should be rotated to prevent bottlenecks and interruption in workflow. Adequate time should be available to permit re-equilibration of the incubator following cleaning, to verify adequate temp and pH, prior to re-introducing patient samples.

- Wear gloves.
- Empty water pan if present.

- Remove all internal components (walls, shelves, inserts, etc.).
- Components should be wiped with the appropriate low-VOC agent. Common approaches include use of a dilution laboratory detergent, followed by rinsing with sterile, purified water. A final wipe with hydrogen peroxide is also recommended. If an autoclave of sufficient size is available, removable components may be autoclaved.
- Wipe and rinse internal walls of incubator thoroughly. Make sure to clean rubber gaskets and other areas around doors.
- Do a final wipe with hydrogen peroxide or low-VOC cleaner.
- Reassemble internal components.
- Replace any filters (hepa, inline, etc.).
- Refill water pan with sterile distilled water if present.
- Record cleaning on the incubator QC paperwork and file in lab records.

Note: Read manufacturer's recommendations on specifics regarding cleaning of other incubator components, such as water jackets.

4

Preparation for Follicle Aspiration and Isolation of Cumulus-Oocyte-Complexes (COC)

Markus Montag

Required Equipment

- Ultrasound device for transvaginal ultrasound
- Transvaginal ultrasound cover
- Ultrasound gel
- Follicle aspiration pump
- Follicle puncture needle
- Tubes for follicle fluid collection (usually 13–15 mL tubes)
- Heating block for tubes [*Optional:* heated transportation device for tube transfer to the laboratory]
- Stereo microscope with heated plate
- Lamina flow hood with build-in heated plate [*Optional:* free-standing heating plate]
- Incubator with appropriate % CO_2/eventually low oxygen (5%–7% O_2)
- Cell culture dishes for follicular aspirate, collection medium and wash medium
- Thermal chips for cell culture dishes
- Pipette equipment for collecting COC (handling pipette/100 μL pipette + tips)
- Gloves (non-powder)
- Documentation chart

To Be Prepared on the Day Before

- Flushing medium for ovum pick up (OPU) [*Optional:* with heparin]
- COC collection medium in a tube for collection and rinsing (5–10 mL HEPES- or MOPS-buffered, warmed overnight at 37°C)
- IVF culture medium in a tube (standard IVF culture media, gassed overnight in an incubator at 37°C)
- Oocyte culture dish with normal IVF culture media/ with or without oil (gassed overnight in an incubator at 37°C) (see Chapter 2)

Preparation on the Day

- Prepare lamina flow hood (for general recommendations see Chapter 2).
- Pre-warm all heating devices to the appropriate temperature.
- Pre-warm sufficient number of tubes (approximately 1 per follicle) for follicular fluid collection (warming incubator/tube heater).
- Make sure that all required material that gets in contact with follicular fluid/COC is properly heated to 37°C.
- Pre-warm cell culture dishes for follicular aspirate (heating plate/warm incubator).
- Place COC collection dish(es) on heated plate of the lamina flow/eventually use thermal chips for direct heat transfer.

Follicle Puncture Assistance

- Double-check patient name and birth date and align with patient files and laboratory.
- Check vacuum/negative pressure at aspiration pump (recommended 150–180 mmHg).
- Check proper fitting of the collection tube to the tube adaptor in the aspiration line.
- During aspiration, give feedback if aspirate is flowing or at hold.
- Note if aspirate comes from left or right ovary.
- Change collection tube if it is filled by 2/3 to 3/4. This is easiest done in a tube heater where tubes are standing side by side by placing the tube adaptor to a new tube.
- Close filled tubes and place into the tube heater at reach for the laboratory or keep warm in tube heater.
- In case of flushing use pre-warmed Flushing medium.

Searching for Cumulus-Oocyte-Complexes

- Wear gloves.
- Identify patient/material provided with patient name.
- Place tubes with follicular fluid in a tube heater close to the stereo microscope.
- Move COC collection dish close to the stereo microscope.
- Fill HEPES-/MOPS-buffered collection medium into collection dish; cover with lid.
- Empty tube with follicular aspirate into 1–2 cell culture dishes.
- Identify COC first by looking from the side, then by checking through the stereo microscope.
- Transfer COC with pipette and little follicular fluid into COC collection dish.
- Do not leave COC too long in pipette (it will have a cooling effect).
- Place dish aside on the heated plate, cover with lid.
- Continue with next tube, and repeat until all tubes are inspected.
- Give regular feedback on how many COC are isolated if location where aspiration is done is close by.
- After all COCs are collected, rinse COCs in collection dish several times. [*Optional:* Use a center-well dish with medium for collection in the center and additional collection medium for rinsing in the outer ring.]
- In case of intense blood contamination, use a second dish for washing with collection medium.
- Remove gassed IVF culture medium from incubator, fill into another pre-warmed dish and rinse COC (alternatively one can use a separate rinsing dish that has been set up on the day before and was properly gassed with extra droplets with IVF medium).
- Remove oocyte culture dish from the incubator and transfer COC into this dish (check patient name or label **now**).
  - For ICSI 8 to 10 COC may be placed in a well with 400–600 μL medium.
  - For IVF up to 4 COC may be placed in a well with 400–600 μL medium or 1 COC per droplet of 50 μL medium.
- Mark the number of COC per well/dish.
- Place dish back into gassed incubator. [*Optional:* Place into a new incubator.]
- Clean work place with non-alcohol agent (e.g., quarternary ammonia).
- Prepare for next OPU.

BIBLIOGRAPHY

Belaisch-Allart, J.C., A. Hazout, F. Guillet-Rosso, M. Glissant, J. Testart, and R Frydman. 1985. "Various Techniques for Oocyte Recovery in an In Vitro Fertilization and Embryo Transfer Program." *Journal of In Vitro Fertilization and Embryo Transfer* 2: 99–104.

Johansson, L. "Handling Gametes and Embryos: Oocyte Collection and Embryo Culture." In *A Practical Guide to Selecting Gametes and Embryos*, edited by M. Montag, 17–38. Taylor & Francis Group, CRC Press, 2014.

Wikland, M. "Oocyte Retrieval." In *In Vitro Fertilization: A Practical Approach*, edited by D.K. Gardner, 120–8. New York: Informa Healthcare USA Inc., 2006.

5

Semen Collection and Sample Reception

Carin Huyser

The first step to collect and evaluate a semen sample can be a daunting experience for male patients.

Circumstances surrounding the production of a semen sample may affect the male and thus the collection and quality of the sample.

Requirements

Location

- Reception area with consultation room, access compliant for physically disabled patients
- Private and comfortable semen collection room(s) with basic washing facilities, where a partner may assist with specimen collection

Equipment and Disposables

- Self-adhesive preprinted labels or permanent markers to indicate unique identifiers, i.e., name, laboratory number and unique codes or other particulars to unequivocally identify the patient and specimen, particulars of investigation required
- Nitrile gloves (non-powder) approved for laboratory use
- Benchtop or mobile incubator in air at 37°C (set temperature as indicated by standard operative procedures)

Collection Containers and Utilities

Standard Collection

- Non-toxic sterile specimen collection container (non-spermicidal plastic vial approved by laboratory) with a tight-fitting lid
- *Optional:*
  - A ziplock-plastic bag to place the specimen container in when transporting the sample from home or when the semen is for decontamination purposes
  - Recyclable eco-friendly cups with lids to hold sample collection containers. The cup

is lightweight and disposable, has insulating properties, keeps the sample vial in an upright position and conceals the contents

Other Optional Collection Aids/ Methods Prescribed by Physician

- A non-spermicidal silastic condom with manufacturer's instructions for collection of a semen sample
- A medically approved vibrator with instructions for vibro-stimulation
- A pre-packed basic kit containing items for sample collection from home or at a different locality outside of the laboratory environment
- A laboratory-approved container with lid to collect a post-ejaculatory urine sample for retrograde ejaculation evaluation

Documentation According to the Laboratory's Specific Protocol

Information/Patient Instructions

- The purpose of semen analysis in laymen's terms (patient brochure)
- A basic stepwise explanation of how to produce a semen sample/use of a silastic condom/ post-ejaculation urine collection for retrograde ejaculation
- Directions to the private semen collection room and spermatology laboratory (if consultation area is not in the vicinity of these areas)

Patient Files and Additional Forms

- Checklist for verbal and written information to be provided or obtained from the patient
- Unique identifiers and personal information forms
- Patient referral letter with contact details for the referring clinician
- Relevant clinical details including previous investigations and screening results of sexually transmitted infection tests

- Informed consent forms for specific investigation/treatment required
- Laboratory spermiogram forms
- Form to note the time of sample production, reception and starting of the analysis, sample spilled and/or problems producing the sample, details of laboratory staff receiving the sample and witness(es) who confirmed the specimen and patient's identification

To Be Prepared the Day Before

- Obtain patient referral and booking information for males who:
  - have been referred for:
    - cryopreservation prior to ART procedure
    - diagnostic or therapeutic sperm analysis and/or processing
    - donation of sperm
    - microbiological analyses of semen
    - post-vasectomy analyses
    - retrograde ejaculation
    - semen decontamination for e.g., HIV/HCV+ patients
  - need home-collection kits
  - require assistance with semen collection, i.e., requested the presence of a partner/prescription medication/vibrator in order to produce a semen sample; be prepared to consult with disabled patients or to accommodate an interpreter
- Either prepare a new file (first visit) or retrieve a previous file (earlier reports)
- Prepare sufficient home-collection kits (*if needed*)
- Ensure the semen collection room(s), toilets and washing basins are neat and clean

Preparation on the Day

- Pre-warm all heating devices/incubators to the appropriate temperature.
- Confirm bookings/cancellations.

General Patient Consultation

- Patient registration should be done prior to consultation, and should be confirmed by the receptionist.
- Obtain the patient's referral letter (filed, placed in patient file or provided by patient).
- Meet, identify and usher patient (or couple) according to the appointment schedule, to the consultation room.
- Use the dedicated checklist in the patient's file to verify that verbal and written information are provided or obtained from the patient:

- Confirm the reason for the appointment.
- Provide an overview of procedures to follow and give the patient time to voice concerns and ask questions.
- Explain that when a chain of custody must be followed, the samples must be produced on-site, i.e., in legal/forensic cases, sperm-banking, donation or assisted reproduction treatment.
- Provide informed consent and documentation according to current regulation and statutory codes of practice:
  - Ensure sufficient time for the patient to read through the documents, ask questions and complete the forms.
  - Co-sign all necessary documentation and assist patients to complete forms where necessary.
- Check the completeness of the patient's form and file.
- Verify sample unique identifiers in the patient's file and the labeled specimen vial.

Issuing Specimen Collection Containers

Provide verbal and written information/patient instructions regarding:

- Abstinence period at the time of semen collection (minimum of 2 days and a maximum of 7 days).
- Avoidance of commensal microbial contamination of the semen sample through urination by the male; washing, rinsing and drying of the genitals and hands and ejaculation into the sterile specimen container.
- The time of sample delivery that should be noted; also, when a sample is collected off-site, transport of the specimen to the laboratory should be within 30 minutes, and at most within 1 h.
- Semen decontamination protocols and procedures when an HIV+ patient is referred to the laboratory.
- The use of non-spermicidal condoms and lubricants, with reference to suitable prescribed products or the availability of laboratory issued embryo tested mineral oil as a lubricant.
- Procedures to follow when:
  - samples will be collected at home and delivered by third parties.
  - retrograde ejaculation is suspected, i.e., if no ejaculate is produced during an orgasm.
  - inability to produce a semen sample by masturbation alone; whereby a home collection with visual aids, alternative reading material, or the use of medically approved vibrator are required.

Receiving Specimens

- Adhere to the laboratory's witnessing procedural protocol to verify that particulars of the patient and sample container, referral and report forms match.
- Reject unlabeled specimens and discard if the identifier codes differ.
- Confirm the recorded date, time of collection, sample reception, and persons who received the sample/ act as witness.
- Indicate if the sample was collected on or off site.
- Note in the report if the sample is incomplete, and if a second sample should be collected.
- Record the duration of sexual abstinence.
- Document recent illnesses or medications prescribed and used.

- Accept the specimen container, and place the vial in a temperature-controlled incubator in air.
- Notify laboratory staff of the specimen to be evaluated and record placement in the incubator.

BIBLIOGRAPHY

Björndahl, L., D. Mortimer, C. Barrat, et al. *A Practical Guide to Basic Laboratory Andrology.* Cambridge: Cambridge University Press, 2010.

Tomlinson, M.J., S.J. Harbottle, B.J. Woodward, and K.S. Lindsay on behalf of the ABA. 2012. "Association of Biomedical Andrologists—Laboratory Guidelines for Good Practice Version 3—2012." *Human Fertility* 15(45): 156–73.

World Health Organization. *Laboratory Manual for the Examination and Processing of Human Semen.* 5th ed. Cambridge: Cambridge University Press, 2010.

6

Spermiogramm, Makler Chamber, Neubauer Chamber, CASA

Verena Nordhoff

Required Equipment

- Stereo microscope with ×20 and ×40 objectives including a heated plate
- Incubator (37°C) without CO_2 when using HEPES or MOPS buffered medium or with 5% CO_2 when using a culture medium
- Round-bottom sterile tubes (e.g., 9 mL or 13 mL tubes)
- Centrifuge (table centrifuge)
- Pipette equipment
- Cell counter
- Heating block
- Counting chamber:
  - Makler chamber
  - Neubauer chamber
  - other disposable chambers for CASA systems
- Gloves (non-powder)
- CASA system
- Lab book and/or computer system or program for documentation

To Be Prepared on the Day Before

- Sperm preparation medium (HEPES- or MOPS-buffered, warmed—eventually gassed)
- WHO-recommended dilution buffer (for use of Neubauer chamber)

Preparation on the Day

- Pre-warm all heating devices to the appropriate temperature.
- Clean the Makler and Neubauer chambers with Aqua Bidest Water and dry well (not necessary in case of disposable chambers e.g., the Leija chamber).
- Store the Makler and Neubauer chamber on a heating device at 37°C.

- Native ejaculate as well as a sperm preparation using either the swim up or the density gradient method (see WHO Manual for exact preparation) can be used for both chambers.
- Keep the sperm preparation sample in the incubator.

Using the Makler Chamber

- **Note:** The Makler chamber is not recommended by WHO for any analysis of a sperm sample, neither for concentration and motility, nor for morphology:
  - Concentration cannot be correctly assessed as the volume evaluated is too low.
  - For motility prepare a wet preparation with 20 μm deepness and examine the three motility categories (progressive [=PR], non-progressive [=NP] and immotile [=IM]) and follow the rules of the WHO Manual 2010.
  - For morphology follow the rules of the WHO Manual 2010 and use the stated staining solutions and the methods described; this is necessary as a neat sample cannot be scored for morphology without a staining!
- Wear gloves.
- Identify patient/material provided with patient name.
- The Makler counting chamber has a thickness of 10 μm and the lid provides a grid with 10 × 10 squares (each square is 100 μm × 100 μm).
- Put a drop of about 5 μL of ejaculate onto the pre-warmed Makler chamber (mix the sample well before adding):
  - If sperm sample is too dense for analysis it is possible to dilute the sample with sperm preparation medium. (**Note:** Take the dilution factor into account when displaying the result.)
- Cover with the corresponding graduated lid (this creates a chamber with sperm in only one layer for better counting).

- Do not wait too long until counting to avoid drying of the sample.
- For measurement of concentration, count the sperm heads (not the tails) in 10 squares of the field, this number X represents the concentration of spermatozoa in millions per milliliter.
  - In case of oligozoospermic samples, count all 100 squares and add to the generated number "00.000", which gives the concentration of spermatozoa per mL.
  - If counting of motile spermatozoa is too difficult, it is possible to immobilize them by placing the sample in hot (60°C) water.
- For motility assessment, first count the number of immotile spermatozoa in a defined number of squares (9–16 in the middle of the grid) and only after that the motile ones in the same squares, and classify them according to WHO categories.
  - Repeat that in several areas for higher reliability.
  - Display the result in % of all counted spermatozoa.
- Document the findings.

Preparation of Neubauer Chamber

- **Note:** The Neubauer chamber can only be used for the analysis of concentration according to WHO Manual 2010, it is not recommended for motility and morphology:
  - For motility prepare a wet preparation with 20 µm deepness and examine the three motility categories (progressive (=PR), non-progressive (=NP) and immotile (=IM)) and follow the rules of the WHO Manual 2010.
  - For morphology follow the rules of the WHO Manual 2010 and use the stated staining solutions and the methods described; this is necessary as a neat sample cannot be scored for morphology without a staining!
- Wear gloves.
- Breath onto the Neubauer chamber and place the cover slip on the middle of the chamber until the Newton's rings are visible (important as otherwise the upper and the lower chamber do not have the correct volume).
- Two chambers, one on the top and one on the bottom are created.
- Identify patient/material provided with patient name.
- Dilute the sperm sample according to WHO recommendation with buffer to fix the sperm for better counting (take this dilution into account when displaying the result).

- Fill 10 µL of fixed sperm each into the upper and the lower chamber.
- Place the Neubauer chamber on a heating block for 2–5 min until the sperm sample has settled (do not wait longer as the sample may dry out).
- Place the chamber on the microscope stage and search for the middle grid (No. 5; for exact picture see WHO Manual).
- Start counting the spermatozoa in grid No. 5; this grid is divided again into 25 squares, each of which has three lines around 16 smaller squares.
- Count only complete spermatozoa with head and tail.
- The location of the head is important, not the location of the tail.
- The boundary of a square is the middle of the three lines.
- Only count the spermatozoon if most of the head lies between the two inner lines.
- Avoid counting the same spermatozoon e.g., by counting sperms on the boundary in a L-shape (meaning only the left and the lower ones lying on the middle line are counted).
- Count at least 200 spermatozoa in the lower and the upper chamber (meaning 2 × 200 spermatozoa).
- Display the finding in the lab book and calculate the final concentration by taking the dilution into account (see table in WHO Manual for correct calculation).

Analysis Using a CASA System

- There are different CASA systems on the market, either they are attached to a standard microscope or they have a built-in microscope.
- Systems can be used for determination of concentration, motility and morphology.
- Start the CASA system and preheat the chamber.
- Equip the chamber proposed by CASA manufacturer with the mandatory volume of the sperm sample.
- Put the corresponding chamber into the machine and run the analysis according to the manufacturer's protocol.
- Display the results and store them on the computer drive. Alternatively, record the results in your lab book.

BIBLIOGRAPHY

World Health Organization. *Laboratory Manual for the Examination of Human Semen*. 5th ed. Cambridge: Cambridge, University Press, 2010.

7

Sperm Viability Testing

Markus Montag

Application Possibilities for Sperm Viability Testing

- Diagnostic sperm assessment in a known case with immotile spermatozoa prior initiation of assisted reproductive treatment
- Testicular biopsy/aspirate with only immotile spermatozoa after preparation
- Epididymal aspirate with only immotile spermatozoa after preparation
- Immotile sperm on the day of assisted reproductive treatment
- Immotile sperm from a retrograde ejaculate preparation

Required Equipment for All Procedures

- Incubator with appropriate % CO_2
- Inverted microscope with micromanipulation equipment, heated stage and 40× lens
- Microinjection capillary
- Suitable culture dishes (ICSI dishes, see Chapter 11)
- Pipette equipment for dish preparation and loading sperm to dish (Serological pipette, 5–10 mL; 1–10 µL pipette + tips)
- HOS medium
- Theophylline
- Laser attached to inverted microscope
- Documentation chart

To Be Prepared on the Day Before

- Culture media for warming overnight (HEPES/ MOPS buffered without gassing)
- Mineral/paraffin oil to be pre-warmed overnight

Preparation on the Day

- Pre-warm all heating devices to the appropriate set-point temperature and control visually that the set-point has been reached.
    - **Note:** An appropriate set-point temperature is the one that gives the correct required temperature in the culture media in a tube or culture dish/requires control.
- Make sure that all material that is used for preparation of the dishes is properly heated to 37°C.
- Pre-warmed/-incubated culture dishes for sperm manipulation (can be used for injection if prepared with PVP and medium droplets for oocytes according to Chapter 11).
- Prepare setup for micromanipulation at the inverted microscope.
- For hypo-osmotic swelling (HOS) test.
    - Prepare HOS medium by mixing HEPES/ MOPS buffered culture medium and bi-distilled water 1:1.
    - Place in a dish: 25–50 µL droplet of HOS medium, 25 µL washing droplet with HEPES/ MOPS buffered medium [*Optional:* PVP and droplets for oocyte injection].
- For sperm flexibility/theophylline/laser test:
    - Prepare a dish with 2–3 × 50 µL droplets and one small 2 µL droplet with HEPES/MOPS buffered medium [*Optional:* PVP and droplets for oocyte injection].

Viability Test by Hypo-Osmotic Swelling Medium

- Pipette a small volume of sperm preparation (<5 µL) into the HOS medium droplet.
- Carefully observe spermatozoa for signs of HOS reaction (refer to WHO Manual or original publications for classification).

- Isolate HOS positive spermatozoa with an injection capillary, aspirating the head first.
- Release spermatozoa in the washing droplet to wash off HOS medium.
- Store spermatozoa in the washing droplet.

Viability Test by Sperm Flexibility Testing

- Pipette a small volume of sperm preparation (<5 μL) into 50 μL droplet, mix gently.
- Touch the sperm tail with an injection capillary and try tail bending. Sperm with a flexible tail have a higher viability chance than others. Stiff tails characterize non-viable spermatozoa.
- Isolate tail-flexible spermatozoa with an injection capillary, aspirating the head first.
- Release spermatozoa in the small collection droplet.

Viability Test Using Theophylline

- Pipette a small volume of sperm preparation (<5 μL) into one 50 μL medium droplet.
- Add 2.5–5 μL theophylline ready to use sperm activation medium, mix gently and incubate at a warm plate for 5 min.
- After 5 min screen droplet for spermatozoa with motility (flickering sperm tail).
- Isolate motile spermatozoa with an injection capillary, aspirate head first.
- Release spermatozoa in the small collection droplet.
- **Note:** Theophylline activity will decrease after 20 to 30 min. If required, use another 50 μL droplet and repeat sperm loading and activation.

Viability Test by Laser

- Pipette a small volume of sperm preparation (<5 μL) into 50 μL droplet, mix gently.
- Switch on the laser.
- Locate the last 1/3 towards the end of the sperm tail to the laser target position.
- Apply a single laser pulse at a pulse length that is half of that required for assisted hatching (alternate: set the laser pulse length to a value that results in a 7–8 μm opening in the zona pellucida of an immature oocyte).

- Carefully observe spermatozoa for a curling reaction at the sperm tail (refer to original publications on laser sperm treatment).
- Isolate reacted spermatozoa with an injection capillary, aspirate head first.
- Release spermatozoa in the small collection droplet.

ICSI with Sperm Identified to Be Viable

- For all tests: Isolate 2–3 spermatozoa more than the number of oocytes for injection.
- Prior ICSI collect spermatozoa from the collection droplet and move to the injection dish. [*Optional:* Place oocytes in injection droplets if the dish was prepared accordingly.]
- **Note:**
  - Viable sperm identified by hypoosmotic swelling dish should be washed in medium prior use for injection.
  - Viable sperm identified by theophylline can be used directly or after washing in a separate medium droplet.
  - Laser-identified viable sperm can be directly used for ICSI.
  - Viable sperm detected by HOS and laser will still be immotile, whereas theophylline will give motile sperm.

BIBLIOGRAPHY

Aktan, T.M., M. Montag, S. Duman, H. Gorkemli, K. Rink, and T. Yurdakul. 2004. "Use of a Laser to Detect Viable but Immotile Spermatozoa." *Andrologia* 36(6): 366–9.

Ebner, T., G. Tews, R.B. Mayer, S. Ziehr, W. Arzt, W. Costamoling, and O. Shebl. 2011. "Pharmacological Stimulation of Sperm Motility in Frozen and Thawed Testicular Sperm Using the Dimethylxanthine Theophylline." *Fertility and Sterility* 96(6): 1331–6.

Nordhoff, V., A.N. Schüring, C. Krallmann, M. Zitzmann, S. Schlatt, L. Kiesel, and S. Kliesch. 2013. "Optimizing TESE-ICSI by Laser-Assisted Selection of Immotile Spermatozoa and Polarization Microscopy for Selection of Oocytes." *Andrology* 1: 67–74.

Ved, S., M. Montag, A. Schmutzler, G. Prietl, G. Haidl, and van der Ven H. 1997. "Pregnancy Following Intracytoplasmic Sperm Injection of Immotile Spermatozoa Selected by the Hypo-Osmotic Swelling-Test: A Case Report." *Andrologia* 29(5): 241–2.

8

Sperm Preparation—Swim Up, Density Gradient, Migration Chamber, Zeta Method

Thomas Ebner

Required Equipment

All Sperm Processing Techniques

- Lamina flow hood [*Optional:* clean workplace]
- Incubator with appropriate temperature and CO_2 [*Optional:* reduced oxygen]
- Sperm washing medium (buffered with HEPES/ MOPS or bicarbonate)
- Surgical gloves (non-powder)
- Syringe with gauge 18 or 19 needle

Swim Up, Density Gradient, Zeta Method

- Centrifuge
- Associated centrifuge tubes

Migration Chamber

- Sterilizable sperm selector [*Optional:* disposable selector]

To Be Prepared the Day Before

All Sperm Processing Techniques

- Pre-warm [*Optional:* and pre-gas] sperm washing medium

Preparation on the Day

All Sperm Processing Techniques

- Clean laminar flow hood with non-alcohol agent. [*Optional:* workplace.]
- Check for seropositivity. [*Optional:* If previous finding is known, choose sperm processing technique.]

Density Gradient

- Place 1 mL of higher density gradient at the bottom of a tube.
- Overlay with 1 mL of lower density gradient. [*Optional:* Underlay lower density with higher density gradient.]
- Pre-warm [*Optional:* and pre-gas] density gradients.

Sperm Preparation

All Sperm Processing Techniques

- Identify patient.
- Provide sterile sperm collection container.
- Wear gloves.
- Keep container at room temperature. [*Optional:* incubator.]
- Control for liquefaction (within 15 minutes). [*Optional:* If liquefaction is delayed (>60 minutes) use mechanical (needle) or enzymatical (bromelain) method to assist.]
- Depending on the method chosen, transfer liquefied ejaculate in tubes or selector. For density gradient overlay the density gradient with liquefied ejaculate.
- Clean working place with non-alcoholic detergent.

Swim Up

- Add 1.5 mL volume of pre-warmed sperm washing medium to specimen. [*Optional:* Make 1:1 dilution with ejaculate.]
- Mix ejaculate-medium suspension with needle for homogenization.
- Centrifuge at 300 g for 8–10 minutes.
- Remove supernatant.
- Resuspend the pellet in 0.5–1 mL of pre-warmed sperm washing medium. [*Optional:* Calculate

number of sperm in pellet and adapt volume of pre-warmed sperm washing medium.]
- Repeat centrifugation step.
- Carefully remove excess supernatant and leave 100–300 μL overlay on pellet (depending on assisted reproductive technology planned).
- Use motile sperms accumulating in supernatant.

Density Gradient

- Place 1 mL of semen above 2 mL of pre-warmed density gradients.
- Centrifuge at 300–400 g for 15–30 minutes.
- Remove most of the supernatant containing density gradient as well as gelatinous bodies and mucus strands.
- Resuspend the sperm pellet in fresh pre-warmed sperm washing medium.
- Centrifuge at 200 g for up to 10 minutes.
- Repeat the last two steps.
- Resuspend pellet of motile sperms for usage.

Zeta Method

- Positively charge a centrifugation tube (e.g., by simply rotating a tube for a couple of times in a latex glove).
- Place native semen in positively charged tube (volume depends on sperm count).
- Allow mature and thus negatively charged sperms to bind to positively charged tube (for 1 minute).
- Centrifuge at 200 g for 10 minutes.
- Invert tube to dispose of non-adhering sperm and other contaminants.
- Rinse the tube with sperm washing medium to collect adhering sperms for usage.

Migration Chamber

- Unwrap sterilized migration chamber [*Optional:* disposable chamber].

- Separately fill migration chamber with liquefied ejaculate and sperm washing medium. Take care that there is no contact between the two compartments.
- Create contact between the two compartments (e.g., placing an insertion ring in the chamber). Take care to do it in a sterile manner.
- Check for contamination of sperm washing medium with native semen.
- Allow sperm to migrate to compartment containing sperm washing medium for 30–60 minutes.
- Interrupt contact between medium (containing accumulated motile spermatozoa) and raw semen.
- Check for motile sperm concentration.
- *Optional:* If dilution of sperms is too high, concentrate them using a centrifugation step at 200 g for 10 minutes.

BIBLIOGRAPHY

Chan, P.J., J.D. Jacobson, J.U. Corselli, and W.C. Patton. 2006. "A Simple Zeta Method for Sperm Selection Based on Membrane Charge." *Fertility and Sterility* 85: 481–6.

Ebner, T., O. Shebl, M. Moser, R.B. Mayer, W. Arzt, and G. Tews. 2011. "Easy Sperm Processing Technique Allowing Exclusive Accumulation and Later Usage of DNA-Strandbreak-Free Spermatozoa." *Reproductive Biomedicine Online* 22: 37–43.

Said, T.M. and J.A. Land. 2011. "Effects of Advanced Selection Methods on Sperm Quality and ART Outcome: A Systematic Review." *Human Reproduction Update* 17: 719–33.

Seiringer, M., M. Maurer, O. Shebl, K. Dreier, G. Tews, S. Ziehr, G. Schappacher-Tilp, E. Petek, and T. Ebner. 2013. "Efficacy of a Sperm-Selection Chamber in Terms of Morphology, Aneuploidy and DNA Packaging." *Reproductive Biomedicine Online* 27: 81–8.

World Health Organization. *Laboratory Manual for the Examination and Processing of Human Semen.* 5th ed. Geneva: WHO Press, 2010.

9

Sperm Selection Using Hyaluronan Binding

Denny Sakkas

Required Equipment

- Stereo microscope with heated plate
- Heating block for dishes
- Pipette equipment for dispensing media, polyvinylpyrrolidone (PVP) and sperm sample (handling pipette/5–20 μL pipette + tips)
- High-powered inverted microscope used for ICSI
- Gloves (non-powder)
- Labeling and recording documentation
- PICSI sperm selection dishes (physiological intracytoplasmic sperm injection—PICSI)
- Soluble hyaluronan solution

Adjunct Protocols

- Sperm preparation protocol
- ICSI protocol

Selection of Sperm

- Identify patient sperm sample, egg dish after hyaluronidase treatment and patient documentation. It is important to perform this technique only on patients who have previously shown low binding to hyaluronan.
- Have dishes, sperm samples and documentation witnessed to confirm that they match.
- Prepare hyaluronan dish (PICSI or soluble hyaluronan solution).

PICSI Dish Preparation

- Place a 10 μL drop of HEPES buffered human tubal fluid (HTF) medium with at least 5 mg/mL of serum protein at the end of each of the three lines on the PICSI dish to hydrate the hyaluronan dots.

- The three hyaluronan dots need to be hydrated at least 5 minutes prior to the procedure.
- Place a PVP drop in the lower part of the dish as a sperm harvesting droplet.
- Optionally, droplets for performing the ICSI procedure can also be placed in the same dish.
- Cover the dish with oil.

Dish Preparation Soluble Hyaluronan Solution

- Place a 10 μL droplet of soluble hyaluronan solution in an elongated shape in the middle of a dish.
- Place an elongated PVP droplet or HEPES buffered medium droplet at 90° facing the middle of the hyaluronan droplet.
- Optionally, droplets for performing the ICSI procedure can also be placed in the same dish.
- Cover the dish with oil.

Sperm Capture PICSI Dish

- Add sperm to one drop, the amount depends on the concentration of the sperm sample to be used. Prior to preparation, check that the concentration is sufficient for sperm selection. To enable a better selection it sometimes helps to vary the sperm concentration in the three drops. Too much sperm can also make selection difficult.
- Allow sperm to incubate for 5–30 minutes, depending on the amount of binding observed.
- Observe the sperm initially after 5 minutes to see if migration to the hyaluronan dot and attachment has already occurred. Set up to perform the ICSI procedure as usual.
- Bound sperm can be identified when they show no progression and their tail beating is vigorous.
- Once an identified bound sperm is located, pick up the bound sperm from the center of the hyaluronan

dot. The head will attach and the tail will be moving in place.

- Place the sperm into the PVP harvesting drop and repeat the process until you have approximately double the amount of sperm than eggs for the ICSI case.

Sperm Capture in Soluble Hyaluronan Solution

- Add sperm to the PVP or medium droplet at the side away from the hyaluronan droplet.
- Connect the PVP/medium droplet with the hyaluronan droplet.
- Allow sperm to incubate for 5–10 minutes, depending on concentration and motility.
- Sperm that entered the hyaluronan droplet and are bound to hyaluronan will show slow forward movement or will be stationary.
- Locate bound sperm, pick up in the micropipette and place into PVP and repeat the process until you have approximately double the amount of sperm than eggs for the ICSI case.

Possible Issues with the PICSI Dish

- Use normal searching criteria when picking sperm for ICSI.
- The longer the sperm incubates in the drop, the more binding there will be. This may, however, lead to too many sperm binding and make it harder to select truly bound sperm.
- Allow low concentration specimens to incubate for a longer period of time if necessary.
- Avoid picking up sperm from the edge of the drop as it is sometimes difficult to identify if they are truly bound.
- Sperm will optimally bind to the hyaluronan dot at 30°C. As temperature increases, swimming vigor increases and the swimming force may overcome binding force.
- Over time and increased temperature, it is possible that the edge of the hyaluronan dot will lift off the dish. The center of the hyaluronan dot will remain attached and sperm will still bind.
- For specimens with very low binding, it is possible that sperm will not bind to the PICSI dish. Allow the sperm to incubate in the dish for a longer period of time until satisfied that no binding is occurring.

Possible Issues with Soluble Hyaluronan Solution

- Prepare the dish properly, in particular the location of the hyaluronan and the PVP/medium droplet to each other.
- The proper concentration of motile sperm is important for ease of working.
- Different degrees of binding can be seen depending on the amount of hyaluronan binding sites at the sperm head. This is reflected by the change in motility, ranging from stationary to slightly forward movement. The best strategy is to watch sperm as they move from the PVP/medium part to the hyaluronan part.

BIBLIOGRAPHY

Huszar, G., C.C. Ozenci, S. Cayli, Z. Zavaczki, E. Hansch, and L. Vigue. 2003. "Hyaluronic Acid Binding by Human Sperm Indicates Cellular Maturity, Viability, and Unreacted Acrosomal Status." *Fertility and Sterility* 79: 1616–24.

Huszar, G., A. Jakab, D. Sakkas, C.C. Ozenci, S. Cayli, E. Delpiano, and S. Ozkavukcu. 2007. "Fertility Testing and ICSI Sperm Selection by Hyaluronic Acid Binding: Clinical and Genetic Aspects." *Reproductive Biomedicine Online* 14: 650–63.

Jakab, A., D. Sakkas, E. Delpiano, S. Cayli, E. Kovanci, D. Ward, A. Revelli, and G. Huszar. 2005. "Intracytoplasmic Sperm Injection: A Novel Selection Method for Sperm with Normal Frequency of Chromosomal Aneuploidies." *Fertility and Sterility* 84: 1665–73.

Parmegiani, L., G.E. Cognigni, S. Bernardi, E. Troilo, W. Ciampaglia, and M. Filicori. 2010. "'Physiologic ICSI': Hyaluronic Acid (HA) Favors Selection of Spermatozoa Without DNA Fragmentation and with Normal Nucleus, Resulting in Improvement of Embryo Quality." *Fertility and Sterility* 93: 598–604.

Worrilow, K.C., S. Eid, D. Woodhouse, M. Perloe, S. Smith, J. Witmyer, K. Ivani, C. Khoury, G.D. Ball, T. Elliot, and J. Lieberman. 2013. "Use of Hyaluronan in the Selection of Sperm for Intracytoplasmic Sperm Injection (ICSI): Significant Improvement in Clinical Outcomes—Multicenter, Double-Blinded and Randomized Controlled Trial." *Human Reproduction* 28: 306–14.

10

IVF—Insemination

Markus Montag

Required Equipment

- Stereo microscope with heated plate
- Lamina flow hood with build-in heated plate [*Optional:* free-standing heating plate]
- Incubator with appropriate % CO_2/eventually low oxygen (5%–7% O_2)
- Pipette equipment for sperm pipetting (1–10 μL pipette + tips)
- Gloves (non-powder)
- Documentation chart

To Be Prepared on the Day Before

- Dish for COC culture with normal IVF culture media/with or without oil (gassed)

Preparation on the Day

- Isolate COC as described (Chapter 4).
- Prepare sperm for insemination as described (Chapter 8).
- Prepare a dish for fertilization check if required (use standard medium or HEPES/MOPS buffered medium depending on work time requirements).
- Prepare a dish for further culture of fertilized oocytes (to be used next day) and place in a gassed incubator (see Chapter 2).
- Pre-warm heated stage at lamina flow bench well in advance.

Insemination of Oocytes with Spermatozoa

- Insemination is best done 3 to 4 hours after isolation of COC.
- Wear gloves.
- Place tube with prepared sperm in a tube holder at the lamina stage.

- Remove culture dish with oocytes from the incubator.
- Identify patient name of the sperm preparation tube and the culture dish holding the oocytes.

Adding Sperm to Oocytes

- Insemination in wells: Add 50,000 to 100,000 motile sperm to one well (400 to 600 μL of medium and maximum of 4 COC) and pipette gently to mix. The total volume of sperm preparation added per well should be less than 25 μL.
- Insemination in droplets: Add 5000 to 10,000 motile sperm to one droplet (50 μL of medium and one COC). The total volume of sperm preparation added should be less than 5 μL.
- Work fast, check motility shortly after sperm were added and move dish back to the incubator immediately after insemination.
- In case of more dishes: Remove one dish at a time from the incubator and inseminate one dish after the other.
- Document insemination in patient data file.

Denudation for Fertilization Check

- Prior denudation check the % of motility of spermatozoa in the fertilization dish.
- Gently remove remaining cumulus cells with a wide denuding capillary (170 μm).
- Note if denudation is difficult/cumulus cells are too firm attached.
- Place denuded oocytes in a separate droplet or in a dish for fertilization check (use normal culture medium if procedure requires less than 2–3 minutes/ use HEPES/MOPS buffered medium if procedure requires longer).
- Check for the number of pronuclei at an inverted microscope using 20× or 40× objectives (as described in Chapter 18).

- In case of short insemination (3–5 h): check for the presence of the 2nd polar body and recheck next day for correct fertilization/presence of 2 pronuclei at 16 to 18 h post insemination.
- Move fertilized oocytes into culture dish for further culture.
- Place dish in a gassed incubator.
- Document fertilization.

BIBLIOGRAPHY

Hall, J., and S. Fishel. 1997. "In Vitro Fertilization for Male Infertility: When and How?" *Baillière's Clinical Obstetrics and Gynaecology* 11: 711–24.

Nel-Themaat, L., T. Elliott, C.C. Chang, G. Wright, and Z.P. Nagy. Conventional IVF Insemination. In *Practical Manual of In Vitro Fertilization: Advanced Methods and Novel Devices*, edited by Z.P. Nagy et al., 297–305. New York: Springer, 2012.

11

ICSI

Thomas Freour

Required Equipment

- Inverted microscope with micromanipulators (three dimensions, hydraulic or electric) and heated plate [*Optional:* inverted microscope under laminar flow and placed on an anti-vibration table]
- Incubator with appropriate % CO_2 [*Optional:* low-oxygen atmosphere (5%–7% O_2)]
- Pre-warmed cell culture dishes (heating plate/warm incubator)
- Pipette equipment for oocytes and spermatozoa handling (Stripper + 130 µm tips, 20 µL and 100 µL pipette + tips)
- Holding and injecting micropipettes
- Documentation chart
- *Optional:* Gloves (non-powder)

To Be Prepared on the Day Before

- PVP or alternative products to slow spermatozoa
- Injection medium/with or without oil (gassed)
- Embryo culture medium for subsequent culture after injection

Preparation on the Day

- Pre-warm all heating devices to the appropriate temperature. [*Optional:* Turn on laminar flow hood in order to stabilize air flow and avoid turbulences.]
- Make sure that all required material that gets in contact with the sperm and oocytes is properly heated to 37°C (or to any temperature allowing a 37°C temperature in culture media).
- Prepare ICSI dish.
- Prepare embryo culture dish. [*Optional:* Rinse all preheated lab ware with specific rinsing medium (or culture medium) before use with gametes.]

Sperm Selection and Immobilization

- *Optional:* wear gloves (non-powder).
- Identify patient/material provided with patient name and birth date according to the most secure procedures.
- Place tube with sperm preparation on the bench and pour a few drops of supernatant in the ICSI dish. Adjust the volume to sperm concentration in order to avoid any delay in finding live sperm. Mix with sperm-slowing viscous solution. [*Optional:* cover with oil.]
- Place one or several mature denuded oocytes in small individual microdrops of injection medium on the opposite side of the dish. Cover with preheated and gassed oil. Great attention should be paid to insuring a rapid but safe workflow, in order to maintain a 37°C temperature in the whole dish, mainly because of the very high sensitivity of oocytes to suboptimal temperature and atmosphere variations rapidly resulting in meiotic spindle disorganization. Depending on the sperm concentration, sperm selection can take various times, and the number of oocytes placed in the dish simultaneously should be adapted.
- Select live spermatozoa according to motility and morphology at 400× magnification.
- *Optional:* Use hyaluronate solution to select mature spermatozoa (PICSI/soluble hyaluron).
- *Optional:* Use very high magnification to select the spermatozoa with the best morphology and the least vacuoles in head cytoplasm (IMSI).
- *Optional:* Use HOS test/laser/activating agents to identify live sperm if only immotile sperm cells are available (see Chapter 7).
- Using the injection pipette's spike perpendicular to spermatozoon axis, aggressively immobilize selected sperm by frank mechanical pressure on the flagellum, allowing membrane permeabilization.
- Avoid touching the centriole close to midpiece, try to press the flagellum in its middle.

- If the cell is broken with head and tail separated, discard it.
- Aspire very gently the sperm cell by the tail in the injection pipette, placing the head very close to the extremity of the injection pipette. [*Optional:* Aspire the sperm cell by the head first. This has been shown to result in same fertilization rates in some studies.]
- Move the pipette to one of the microdrops containing an oocyte.

Intracytoplasmic Injection

- Using the suction force of the holding pipette, hold the oocyte in place with the polar body located at 12 or 6 o'clock. [*Optional:* Use optical system to visualize meiotic spindle.]
- Ideally, the bottom of the oocyte should touch the bottom of the dish. Make sure that the suction force is sufficient to avoid any involuntary movement of the oocyte during sperm injection.
- Focus on the border of oocyte's cytoplasm and close the injection pipette, ensuring that both pipettes and sperm are in the same focal plan.
- Push very gently and straight the injection pipette throughout the zona pellucida and then keep moving it forward in a continuous movement until contact with the cytoplasmic membrane. The latter will deform and resist because of its elasticity, until it suddenly breaks when the pipette approximately reaches the center of the cell, allowing the pipette to really enter the cytoplasm, still with the same continuous movement.
- Following membrane breaking, a small amount of cytoplasmic content can eventually move inside the injection pipette, and should be very gently put back in the cytoplasm. This aspiration followed by ejection of some cytoplasmic content is beneficial for fertilization.
- Move the extremity of the pipette approximately to the center of the ooplasm. If the membrane sort of sticks to the injection pipette, move further than the center of the ooplasm in order to allow the membrane to recover its initial shape, but absolutely avoid touching the opposite side of the ooplasm.
- Gently eject the spermatozoon, making sure that it has entirely gone out of the pipette.
- Move the pipette back out of the ooplasm very gently, making sure that the spermatozoon remains in place in the cytoplasm and does not stick to the pipette while it is withdrawn.
- The oocyte should obviously not move at all during the whole procedure, except if focal plan is not correct.
- Free oocyte from holding pipette.
- Using conventional pipette and tips, move oocytes to embryo culture dish, either in individual microdrops or in grouped culture wells.
- Check once again patient name and place dish back into gassed incubator. [*Optional:* Switch to new incubator.]
- Redo the same setup and procedures if some other oocytes remain to be microinjected. [*Optional:* When a series of oocytes is finished, new oocytes from the same cohort can be placed in the same dish using the same injection medium microdrops and the same sperm suspension. However, this should only be considered if procedure is fast enough and performed in sufficiently controlled temperature and atmosphere conditions to allow stable environment throughout the whole process. Covering dish with oil helps in stabilizing temperature and atmosphere within culture medium. Alternatively, prepare several ICSI dishes in order to shorten oocytes' exposure to suboptimal culture conditions while out of the incubator.]
- Once the procedure is complete, clean the microscope and bench with embryo-tested non-alcohol agent.
- Prepare for next ICSI.

BIBLIOGRAPHY

Dumoulin, J.C.M. et al. 2001. "Embryo Development and Chromosomal Anomalies After ICSI: Effect of the Injection Procedure." *Human Reproduction* 16(2): 306–12.

Gardner, D.K., A. Weissman, C.M. Howles, and Z. Shoham. *Textbook of Assisted Reproductive Technologies*, 4th ed. Boca Raton, FL: CRC Press, 2012.

Joris, H. et al. 1998. "Intracytoplasmic Sperm Injection: Laboratory Setup and Injection Procedure." *Human Reproduction* 13(S1): 76–86.

Woodward, B.J. et al. 2008. "A Comparison of Headfirst and Tailfirst Microinjection of Sperm at Intracytoplasmic Sperm Injection." *Fertility and Sterility* 89(3): 711–14.

12

Oocyte In Vitro Maturation—Isolation of COCs and Culture for Maturation

Mariabeatrice Dal Canto and Giovanni Coticchio

Principles

- This procedure concerns the recovery of cumulus cell-oocyte complexes (COCs) found in the follicular fluid collected from women undergoing oocyte in vitro maturation (IVM) treatment.
- Depending on whether women are exposed to mild FSH priming and/or hCG trigger, oocytes may be collected at different maturation stages and therefore may require different culture conditions and times of maturation before insemination by ICSI.
- For such a reason, the different types of COCs should be cultured separately as soon as they are identified and collected from the follicular fluid.

Equipment and Materials

- Laminar flow hood or IVF chamber with built-in stereo microscope and heated working surface
- Heating block for tubes
- 37°C incubator with 5% CO_2/95% atmospheric air
- IVM medium
- HEPES-buffered Flushing medium
- r-FSH stock solution (7.5 IU/mL)
- hCG stock solution (100 IU/mL)
- Center-well and 4-well cell culture dishes
- 60 mm Petri dishes
- 35 mm Petri dishes
- 15 mL conical tubes
- 50 mL flasks
- Pasteur pipette
- 20 mL syringes
- 70 μm cell strainer
- P100 pipette and sterile tips
- Powder-free gloves
- Documentation material

Preparation on the Day before Recovery (Day −2)

- Pre-equilibrate in the incubator the IVM medium supplemented with synthetic serum.

Preparation on the Morning of the Day of Recovery (Day −1)

- For each milliliter of pre-equilibrated protein-supplemented IVM medium, add 10 μL of r-FSH stock solution (7.5 IU/mL) and 1 μL of hCG stock solution (100 IU/mL). This medium will be referred to as "final IVM medium".
- For each IVM oocyte pick-up scheduled on the day, dispense the supplemented IVM medium in a center-well dish (500 μL) and a 4-well dish (500 μL per well). The center-well and 4-well dishes will be used to culture separately expanded and compact COCs, respectively. In case the patient has not been exposed to hCG, expanded COCs will not be collected and therefore preparation of the center-well dish will not be required. Once prepared, place the center-well and the 4-well dishes in the incubator until use.
- Supplement the Flushing medium with heparin (20 IU/mL final concentration), dispense in two 50 mL flasks (one for each ovary), and warm at 37°C. This medium will be required for collecting the follicular fluid.

COC Collection (Day −1)

- Mark materials with patient identification name/code and make sure that this corresponds to the patient name.

- Give the flask containing the heparin-supplemented Flushing medium to the staff assisting the clinician in the oocyte pick-up procedure.
- As soon as follicular aspirates (contained in 50 mL flasks) are delivered from the operating theatre, prepare a 35 mm Petri dish with 2 mL of Flushing medium overlaid with 2 mL of mineral oil. This dish will be referred to as "washing dish".
- Fill two 20 mL syringes with heparin-supplemented Flushing medium.
- Filter the material contained in a collection flask through the strainer, then wash the material retained by the strainer with 2–3 mL of heparin-supplemented Flushing medium.
- Place the strainer overturned in a 60 mm Petri dish. Wash the walls and bottom of the strainer with heparin-supplemented Flushing medium contained in one of the two syringes.
- Repeat the above washing step after placing the strainer in another Petri dish and check through the stereo microscope that all the material has been released from the strainer.
- Observe through the stereo microscope the material released into the 60 mm dishes, identify the COCs and move them to the washing dish.
- Repeat the above steps to collect the material contained in a second 50 mL flask, if appropriate.
- Transfer expanded and compact COCs in pre-equilibrated final IVM Medium contained in a center-well and a 4-well dish, respectively.
- Place the dishes in the incubator and culture expanded and compact COCs for 6 hours and 30 hours of maturation, respectively.
- Take note of number and types of collected oocytes, as well as the time of pick-up and the start time of maturation.

- After 6 and 30 hours of maturation, respectively, manipulate enzymatically and mechanically expanded and compact COCs to release oocytes from surrounding cumulus cells. Carry out this step according to the procedure normally used in ICSI cycles.
- Shortly after cumulus cell removal, inseminate by ICSI morphologically normal oocytes showing an extruded polar body. The above procedure implies that mature oocytes derived from expanded COCs will be microinjected on day −1, whereas in vitro matured oocytes obtained from compact COCs will be microinjected on day 0.
- Carry out the steps following in vitro maturation (ICSI, fertilization check, embryo culture, etc.) according to the procedures normally applied in ICSI cycles.

BIBLIOGRAPHY

Dal Canto, M., F. Brambillasca, M. Mignini Renzini, G. Coticchio, M. Merola, M. Lain, E. De Ponti, and R. Fadini. 2012. "Cumulus Cell-Oocyte Complexes Retrieved From Antral Follicles in IVM Cycles: Relationship Between Cocs Morphology, Gonadotropin Priming and Clinical Outcome." *Journal of Assisted Reproduction and Genetics* 29: 513–19.

Fadini, R., M.B. Dal Canto, M. Mignini Renzini, F. Brambillasca, R. Comi, D. Fumagalli, M. Lain, M. Merola, R. Milani, and E. De Ponti. 2009. "Effect Of Different Gonadotrophin Priming on IVM of Oocytes From Women with Normal Ovaries: A Prospective Randomized Study." *Reproductive Biomedicine Online* 19: 343–51.

13

Artificial Oocyte Activation

Markus Montag

Important Notes

- Artificial oocyte activation (AOA) may help to overcome complete fertilization failure or very low fertilization rates diagnosed in a previous ICSI treatment cycle.
- AOA mimics the initial rise of intracellular calcium that is triggered in human by sperm PLCzeta but not the oscillations that are part of physiological oocyte activation.
- A sperm-derived deficiency in oocyte activation can be assessed by a mouse oocyte activation test.
- A low or absent fertilization in a previous standard IVF cycle is no indication to perform AOA.
- The technique should not be used in standard IVF insemination or in an attempt to enhance the overall fertilization rate.
- The currently applied protocols are considered as experimental and the patient has to give informed consent.

Required Equipment

- Lamina flow hood with build-in stereo microscope and heated plate or free-standing stereo microscope with heated stage
- Incubator with appropriate % CO_2/eventually low oxygen (5%–7% O_2)
- Pre-incubated cell culture dishes for oocyte activation (gassed incubator)
- Pre-incubated cell culture dishes for further culture (gassed incubator)
- Pipette equipment for dish preparation
- Artificial oocyte activation solution (preferentially ready-to-use solution)
- Equipment for oocyte handling
- Gloves (non-powder) according to clinic policy
- Documentation chart

To Be Prepared on the Day Before

- Mineral oil to be pre-warmed overnight
- Cell culture dishes for culture after ICSI and AOA (gassed incubator)

Preparation on the Day

- Pre-warm all heating devices to the appropriate set-point temperature and control visually that the set-point has been reached.
- **Note:** An appropriate set-point temperature is the one that gives the correct required temperature in the culture media in a tube or culture dish/requires control.
- Make sure that all material that is used for preparation of the dishes is properly heated to 37°C.
- Prepare the oocyte activation dish 4–6 h prior to use: 2 droplets of AOA solution (30–50 μL each) and 6 droplets of culture medium for washing (30–50 μL droplets each) and cover with pre-warmed oil/incubate in CO_2 atmosphere for at least 4 h.
- Label with patient name after preparation or next day prior to use.

Oocyte Activation with a Ready-To-Use Calcium Ionophore Solution (A23187)

- AOA is performed immediately after ICSI.
- After ICSI, place the ICSI dish on the heated stage of the stereo microscope.
- Remove the oocyte activation dish from the incubator and place beside the ICSI dish.
- Transfer oocytes with a handling pipette from the ICSI dish into the first AOA droplet in the oocyte activation dish.
- Pipette in and out and immediately place oocytes into the second AOA droplet.

- Place the oocyte activation dish for 10–15 minutes in an incubator with CO_2 atmosphere.
- Remove dish after 10–15 min and place on the heated stereo microscope stage.
- Fill the handling pipette with little medium volume from one of the washing droplets.
- Blow medium over the oocytes, take oocytes into handling pipette and wash thoroughly in the culture media wash droplets in the same dish.
- Remove standard culture dish from the incubator.
- Transfer the oocytes into the standard culture dish for culture after ICSI (check patient name on prepared dish or label **now**).
- Mark the number of oocytes per well/dish.
- Place dish in an incubator with CO_2 atmosphere and culture as usual until fertilization check at 16–18 h after ICSI.
- If required, clean stage with non-alcohol agent (e.g., quaternary ammonia).

Important Notes

- One oocyte activation dish can be used for 12 to 16 oocytes at one time.
- The oocyte activation dish should only be used once and for one patient only.
- If the time needed to inject all oocytes from one patient exceeds 30 minutes, the first batch of oocytes should be activated within 30 min after injection of the first oocyte.
- If more oocytes/more activation rounds are to be done, prepare as many oocyte activation dishes as required.
- AOA will not necessarily result in fertilization rates that are as high as with standard ICSI cases.
- If despite AOA all oocytes are not fertilized, it is very likely that the underlying problem is related to a deficiency within the oocyte that cannot be overcome by AOA. This can only be assessed prior therapy by a mouse oocyte activation test (MOAT) with the sperm or a sperm extract.

Modified Protocols

- AOA was also described by using ionomycin activation solution using a stock solution (1 mmol/L of ionomycin in cell culture tested DMSO) that was diluted immediately prior to use to 10 μM with pre-incubated cell culture medium.
- AOA with ionomycin is performed in two consecutive steps: a first activation procedure is done 30 min after ICSI with a 10 min incubation period in the ionomycin activation solution followed 30 min later by a second activation for another 10 min.
- Handling of oocytes before, during and after each activation step is done as outlined with the standard ready-to-use calcium ionophore solution.

BIBLIOGRAPHY

Ebner, T., M. Köster, O. Shebl, M. Moser, H. Van der Ven, G. Tews, and M. Montag. 2012. "Application of A Ready-to-Use Calcium Ionophore Increases Rates of Fertilization and Pregnancy in Severe Male Factor Infertility." *Fertility and Sterility* 98: 1432–37.

Ebner, T., M. Montag, Oocyte Activation Study Group, M. Montag, K. Van der Ven, H. Van der Ven, T. Ebner, O. Shebl, P. Oppelt, J. Hirchenhain, J. Krüssel, B. Maxrath, C. Gnoth, K. Friol, J. Tigges, E. Wünsch, J. Luckhaus, A. Beerkotte, D. Weiss, K. Grunwald, D. Struller, and C. Etien. 2015. "Live Birth After Artificial Oocyte Activation Using a Ready-to-Use Ionophore: A Prospective Multicentre Study." *Reproductive Biomedicine Online* 30: 359–65.

Ebner, T., P. Oppelt, M. Wöber, P. Staples, R.B. Mayer, U. Sonnleitner, S. Bulfon-Vogl, I. Gruber, A.E. Haid, and O. Shebl. 2015. "Treatment with Ca^{2+} Ionophore Improves Embryo Development and Outcome in Cases with Previous Developmental Problems: A Prospective Multicenter Study." *Human Reproduction* 30: 97–102.

Montag, M., M. Köster, K. van der Ven, U. Bohlen, and H. van der Ven. 2012. "The Benefit of Artificial Oocyte Activation is Dependent on the Fertilization Rate in a Previous Treatment Cycle." *Reproductive Biomedicine Online* 24: 521–6.

Vanden Meerschaut, F., L. Leybaert, D. Nikiforaki, C. Qian, B. Heindryckx, and P. De Sutter. 2013. "Diagnostic and Prognostic Value of Calcium Oscillatory Pattern Analysis for Patients with ICSI Fertilization Failure." *Human Reproduction* 28: 87–98.

14

Cryopreservation—Sperm TESE and MESA

Borut Kovačič

Required Equipment for Cryopreservation/Thawing

- Stereo microscope in laminar flow hood
- Printer for self-adhesive labels
- Sealing system for straws and tubes (Syms III, CryoBioSystem, France)
- Handling forceps
- Liquid nitrogen vessel with holder for straws/tubes [*Optional:* Programmable slow freezing system for controlled cooling]
- Cryogenic storage tank

Preparation on the Day of Cryopreservation

- CBS (CryoBioSystem, France) high-security tubes for testicular samples
- CBS high-security 0.5 mL straws with filling nozzles for epididymal samples
- Suction device for straws
- Visotubes and goblets for CBS straws or cryocanes for CBS tubes
- ICSI Petri dishes
- Test tubes (5 mL)
- Pasteur pipettes (3 mL with large opening)
- Scalpels (bigger size)
- Gloves (non-powder)
- HEPES- or MOPS-buffered sperm preparation medium (SPM) at room temperature
- Paraffin oil
- Sperm cryopreservation medium (CPM) at room temperature
- Fixative solution (e.g., Bouin's fixative)
- Documentation

Preparation of Testicular Tissue

- Check patient's serological tests.
- Wear gloves.
- Immediately after surgery the tissue should be placed into a tube with 1 mL of SPM and labelled appropriately with patient's data.
- When more pieces of tissue were taken, process each piece separately.
- Pour out the content of the tube into the Petri dish.
- In case of a bloody sample, transfer tissue in another dish with fresh SPM (approximately 0.5–1 mL).
- Use a scalpel and cut a small piece of tissue, transfer it into the tube with Bouin's fixative for cytopathological examination and mark the tube with patient's data.
- Using a pair of scalpels, shred and mince a tissue into as small pieces as possible and squeeze them between two scalpels.
- Aspirate nearly all tissue/cell suspension from a dish by using Pasteur pipette and transfer it into a test tube.
- Cover the remaining suspension in a Petri dish with paraffin oil and assess it for the presence of sperm on the microscope at magnification of 200×.
- Evaluate the sperm concentration per microscope field of view (e.g., 1 sperm per five fields), sperm morphology (normal/amorphous), maturity (presence of sperm tail, cytoplasmic droplets) and motility (yes/no).

Preparation of Epididymal Sample

- Check patient's serological tests.
- Wear gloves.
- The epididymal aspirate should be collected directly into SPM.
- Take a droplet of the sample and assess it on microscope for the presence of sperm and their motility.
- Centrifuge the remaining sample at 300 g × 10 min.
- Discard the supernatant and resuspend the pellet in 0.5–1 mL of fresh SPM.

Cryopreservation

- Prepare labels with date, patient and sample data (or code) and stick them on CBS straws or tubes.
- Measure volume of testicular or epididymal sample.
- In a test tube with sperm solution slowly add (it should take 2–5 min) the CPM (drop-wise with swirling) in a ratio 1:1 or 0.75:1 (see manufacturer's recommendation).
- For epididymal sample, connect 0.5 mL CBS straw to the syringe and fill the straw through a filling nozzle.
- For testicular sample, fill CBS tubes with a small volume of testicular sample.
- If possible, prepare more straws or tubes from one biopsy/aspiration.
- Seal straws or tubes by sealer.
- Place a straw/tube holder in the vessel and fill the vessel with liquid nitrogen to the level a couple of centimeters below the level of straw/tube holder.
- Place straws or tubes on a holder for 20 min, then plunge them into liquid nitrogen. [*Optional:* Prepare programmable freezing system and cool the samples.]
- Ramp 1: cooling from 22°C to 4°C with the rate −5°C/min.
- Ramp 2: cooling from +4°C to −80°C with the rate −10°C/min without seeding.
- Ramp 3: rapid cooling (free fall) from −80°C to −160°C.
- Ramp 4: plunge straws/tubes into the liquid nitrogen.
- Using forceps, place the CBS straws in visotubes with the same patient's code and place them into the storage tank. The CBS tubes should be mounted in a cryo cane and moved into the storage tank.
- Fill patient documentation (date, identification code, number of straws/tubes, visotube color, position in the canister/storage tank).

Preparation on the Day of Thawing

- Autoclavable sterile scissors
- ICSI Petri dishes
- 5 mL test tubes
- Pasteur pipettes
- Water bath (37°C)
- Hypochlorite solution
- Sterile water
- SPM
- Paraffin oil
- *Optional:* Sperm motility-enhancing chemicals (e.g., pentoxifylline or CE-marked SpermMobile with theophylline, Gynemed, Germany)

Thawing

- Identify the location of straw/tube in the cryotank and verify color, name or identification code of the frozen sample with data in patient's documentation (double control is highly recommended).
- Prepare water bath to 37°C.
- Move the straw/tube from liquid nitrogen into the water bath for 10 min.
- Wipe the straw/tube with sterile hypochlorite solution, wash it with sterile water and dry it with sterile gauze.
- Cut one end of the straw/tube with sterile scissors and transfer the content to the test tube.
- Put a small drop of the sample into Petri dish and cover with paraffin oil.
- Check for the presence of sperm and motility under microscope at 200× magnification.
- Slowly dilute the remaining thawed sample by adding SPM (5–10× volume of the sample).
- Wash the sample by centrifugation at 500 g × 10 min, discard the supernatant and resuspend the pellet.
- Prepare a dish for ICSI. [*Optional:* Isolate sperm directly from the thawed sample by micromanipulation and transfer them into PVP before ICSI.]
- In case of total sperm immotility, add sperm motility-enhancing solution.

BIBLIOGRAPHY

Gil-Salom, M., J. Romero, Y. Minguez, C. Rubio, M.J. De los Santos, J. Remohí, and A. Pellicer. 1996. "Pregnancies after Intracytoplasmic Sperm Injection with Cryopreserved Testicular Spermatozoa." *Human Reproduction* 11: 1309–13.

Kovačič, B., V. Vlaisavljević, and M. Reljič. 2006. "Clinical Use of Pentoxifylline for Activation of Immotile Testicular Sperm Before ICSI in Patients with Azoospermia." *Journal of Andrology* 27: 45–52.

Mahadevan, M. and A.D. Trounson. 1983. "Effect of Cryoprotective Media and Dilution Methods on the Preservation of Human Spermatozoa." *Andrologia* 15: 355–66.

Verheyen, G., De Croo I, H. Tournaye, I. Pletincx, P. Devroey, and A.C. van Steirteghem. 1995. "Comparison of Four Mechanical Methods to Retrieve Spermatozoa From Testicular Tissue." *Human Reproduction* 10: 2956–9.

15

Vitrification—Oocytes, 2PN, Embryos, Blastocysts

Ana Cobo and Aila Coello

Principles

- Vitrification is a cryopreservation procedure by which an aqueous solution is solidified into a glassy phase without ice crystal formation by applying high cooling rates and increasing viscosity.
- The main shortcoming of the technique is the use of a high concentration of cryoprotectants, which can damage oocytes and embryos through chemical toxicity and osmotic stress.
- New improvements allow reducing toxicity and supporting high cooling rates by using very small volumes.
- The procedure described below is that developed for Cryotop. However, different methods exist on the market and it is advisable to follow the manufacturer's recommendations.

Required Equipment

- Cryotop (Kitazato Biopharma, Tokyo, Japan)
- Repro Plate (Kitazato Biopharma, Tokyo, Japan)
- Cooling rack (styrene box for liquid nitrogen)
- Liquid nitrogen
- Storage tank
- Stereo microscope, stopwatch or timer, tweezers, Pasteur pipette, micropipettes and tips

Solutions

- Basic solution (BS) is made of HEPES-buffered TCM-199 supplemented with hydroxypropyl cellulose (HPC). Only for oocytes vitrification.
- Equilibration solution (ES) consists of 7.5% ethylene glycol (EG) and 7.5% dimethylsulphoxide (DMSO) dissolved in BS.
- Vitrification solution (VS) consists of 15% EG, 15% DMSO and 0.5M trehalose dissolved in BS.
- Thawing solution (TS) consists of 1.0M trehalose dissolved in WS.
- Dilution solution (DS) consists of 0.5M trehalose dissolved in WS.
- Washing solution (WS) is made of HEPES-buffered TCM-199 supplemented with HPC.

Vitrification Process

Preparation on the Day

- Bring BS, ES and VS to room temperature (24°C–26°C) 1 hour before application.
- Fill the cooling rack completely with liquid nitrogen.
- Write necessary information about the patient on the handle of the vitrification device.

Equilibration Step

Differential procedures are applied for oocytes and embryos.

For Oocytes

- Drop 20 μL BS into first well and 300 μL VS each into 2nd and 3rd well of the Repro Plate.
- Place the oocytes (up to 16) with minimal volume of medium at the bottom of BS well. Compare the width of perivitelline space with the thickness of zona pellucida and record it.
- Add 20 μL ES surrounding the previous BS drop. Wait for 3 minutes.
- Add another 20 μL ES gently and wait for 3 minutes.
- Add 240 μL ES gently and wait for 6–9 minutes. The volume of the oocytes is required to recover completely.

For 2PN, Cleavage Stage and Blastocysts

- Drop 300 μL ES into first well and 300 μL VS each into 2nd and 3rd well of the Repro Plate.
- Place the embryo with minimal volume of medium at the top center of ES.

- Equilibration time is as follows:
  - 2PN and embryos: 10–12 min.
  - Blastocysts: 12–15 min.

Vitrification Step

The procedure is the same for oocytes and embryos.

- Place the oocytes/embryos on the surface of VS. Aspirate the remaining ES surrounding them and throw it out of the well. Place the oocytes/embryos at the bottom of the well and continue removing the remaining ES around them changing their position. All this process must be done in 30 seconds.
- Place the oocytes/embryos at the bottom of the 2nd VS well. For a period of 30 seconds, move them throughout the well and remove the surrounding solution.
- Carry the oocytes/embryos at the tip of the pipette and place them on the device strip with minimum volume. Aspirate the excess of solution minimizing the VS drop. No more than four oocytes or two embryos per device must be loaded.
- Plunge the device directly into liquid nitrogen and move it quickly. Keep the device under liquid nitrogen and cover it with the straw cap.

Warming Process

Preparation on the Day

- Warm TS vial and a Petri dish up to 37°C at least 1 hour.
- Bring DS and WS to room temperature (24°C–26°C) 1 hour before application.
- Fill the cooling rack completely with liquid nitrogen and retrieve the device from the storage tank. Keep it submerged in liquid nitrogen.

Dilution and Warming Step

The procedure is the same for oocytes and embryos.

- Remove the cover straw from the device under liquid nitrogen. Drop 300 µL DS into first well and 300 µL WS each into 2nd and 3rd well of the Repro Plate.
- Pour the full content of TS into the Petri dish. Immerse the device into TS situated on the microscope stage with a fast movement. Do not try to recover the oocytes/embryos before 40 seconds.
- After 1 minute immersion in TS, aspirate the oocytes/embryos and take 1 cm of TS.
- Blow TS from the pipette directly to the bottom of the DS well. Place the oocytes/embryos into the TS layer. Wait for 3 minutes.

- Aspirate the oocytes/embryos in DS and load 1 cm of DS. Blow DS to the bottom of the WS1 well and place the oocytes/embryos into the DS layer. Wait for 5 minutes.
- Aspirate the oocytes/embryos with the minimal volume of WS and transfer them to the top center of WS2. After the oocytes/embryos freefall to the bottom of WS2, repeat the process in WS2.
- After 1 minute in WS2, transfer the oocytes/embryos to a culture dish containing the appropriate culture medium. Incubate them at 37°C.

Storage

- Vapor-phase nitrogen freezers are recommended to use for storage.
- Although the use of traditional liquid nitrogen tanks is also allowed, stricter safety measures should be taken during storage and retrieval of the samples in/from the liquid nitrogen tank as these tanks do not provide a working area on which the samples can be manipulated at storage temperatures.
- In all cases, special care should be taken to maintain the samples submerged in liquid nitrogen while moving them from one container to another in order to avoid any change of temperature which can provoke accidental devitrification.

Notes of Caution

- Oocytes should be vitrified within 2 hours after collection.
- ICSI should be performed within 2 hours after warming.

BIBLIOGRAPHY

Cobo, A., M.J. de los Santos, D. Castello, P. Gamiz, P. Campos, and J. Remohi. "Outcomes of Vitrified Early Cleavage-Stage and Blastocyst-Stage Embryos in a Cryopreservation Program: Evaluation of 3,150 Warming Cycles." *Fertility and Sterility* 98: 1138–46.e1.

Cobo, A., M. Meseguer, J. Remohi and A. Pellicer. 2010. "Use of Cryo-Banked Oocytes in an Ovum Donation Programme: A Prospective, Randomized, Controlled, Clinical Trial." *Human Reproduction* 25: 2239–46.

Rienzi, L., S. Romano, L. Albricci, R. Maggiulli, A. Capalbo, E. Baroni, S. Colamaria, F. Sapienza and F. Ubaldi. 2010. "Embryo Development of Fresh 'Versus' Vitrified Metaphase II Oocytes After ICSI: A Prospective Randomized Sibling-Oocyte Study." *Human Reproduction* 25: 66–73.

Yavin, S. and A. Arav. 2007. "Measurement of Essential Physical Properties of Vitrification Solutions." *Theriogenology* 67: 81–9.

16

Slow Freezing: Principles, Oocytes, 2PN, Embryos, Blastocysts

Etienne Van den Abbeel

Principles

- For most mammalian cells including oocytes and embryos, the non-osmotic volume has been calculated as being approximately 20%. In other words, about 80% of the volume of cells is water.
- Cryobiology deals with the fate of this water as the temperature is lowered to temperatures below freezing point. The challenge to cells during freezing is not their ability to endure storage at very low temperatures (less than −180°C); rather, it is the lethality of an intermediate zone of temperature (−15°C to −60°C) that a cell must traverse twice (once during the cooling cycle and once during warming).
- During slow freezing of cells, after loading them with cryoprotectant, at a certain temperature below 0°C extracellular ice crystal formation is induced. As a result, the concentration of salt in the extracellular milieu is increased and the cell osmotically responds and starts to dehydrate.
- When the cells are further cooled slowly enough (at 0.3°C/min) to temperatures between −30°C and −40°C, the cell reaches quasi-equilibrium and there is no risk for intracellular ice crystal formation upon plunging into liquid nitrogen.
- For thawing, the cell must be thawed rapidly (>300°C/min) in order to avoid intracellular recrystallization.

Required Equipment—Materials

- Stereo microscope with heated plate
- Stereo microscope without heated plate
- Laminar air flow hood with free-standing heating plate
- Incubator at 37°C with appropriate CO_2 and reduced oxygen concentration
- Pipette equipment for oocyte and embryo handling

- Cell culture dishes for handling and culture of oocytes and embryos
- Oocyte and embryo culture media also containing human serum albumin (0.5% w/v) (bicarbonate buffered), hereafter referred to as "culture medium"
- Oocyte and embryo handling media also containing human serum albumin (0.5% w/v) (HEPES/MOPS buffered), hereafter referred to as "collection medium"
- Freezing media containing 1.5 mol/L 1.2-propanediol (oocyte, 2PN and embryo freezing) or glycerol (blastocyst freezing) made up in collection media (hereafter referred to as "freezing media A")
- Freezing media containing 1.5 mol/L 1.2-propanediol (oocyte, 2PN and embryo freezing) or glycerol (blastocyst freezing) with 0.2 mol/L sucrose or trehalose made up in collection media (hereafter referred to as "freezing media B")
- Thawing media containing preferentially 0.5, 0.2 mol/L sucrose or trehalose made up in collection media (hereafter referred to as "thawing media A" and "thawing media B" respectively) (these solutions can vary according to commercial companies' formulations)
- Collection, freezing and thawing media should be stored in the refrigerator at 4°C
- Biological freezer
- 37°C warm waterbath
- Seeding forceps (for extracellular ice crystal induction
- Dewar
- Liquid nitrogen
- Liquid nitrogen storage containers
- Protective gloves
- Freezing straws (0.25–0.30 cc)
- Equipment for patient identification on culture dishes and straws
- Mineral/paraffin oil

Standard Freezing Procedure for Oocytes—2PN—Embryos—Blastocysts

Preparations on the Day (One to Two Hours Before Freezing Cells)

- Take out collection and freezing media from the refrigerator (4°C) and equilibrate them at 22°C–26°C.
- Prepare culture dishes containing eight 25 µL droplets of collection medium under oil and keep at 37°C.
- Label plastic freezing straws with the correct patient and cell identification.

Procedure

- For each patient, take the culture dish(es) out of the incubator, identify cells to be frozen in the culture dish under the microscope with heating stage, pipette them into a culture dish containing 25 µL droplets of collection medium (one cell/droplet) under oil at 37°C.
- Bring the culture dish containing the cells at 22°C–26°C for 10 minutes.
- Pipette the cells into freezing medium A and equilibrate for 10–15 minutes at 22°C–26°C.
- Pipette the cells into freezing medium B and equilibrate for 5 minutes at 22°C–26°C.
- Load the cell(s) with freezing medium B in the plastic freezing straws. The cells with freezing medium B are positioned between two air bubbles separating the cells from freezing medium B without cells.
- Heat seal the freezing straw(s) and position the straw(s) in the biological freezer pre-programmed for slow freezing.
- The temperature in the biological freezer is lowered from 22°C to −7°C at 2°C/min, at which temperature a 10 min pre-seeding hold is programmed. Seeding is then performed manually by touching the straws with a liquid nitrogen (LN_2) cold forceps at the level of a 5 mm air bubble. The temperature is then lowered to −30°C at 0.3°C/min, to −150°C at 50°C/min, and straws are then plunged into LN_2.
- Position the freezing straws into liquid nitrogen storage containers.

Standard Thawing Procedure for Oocytes—2PN—Embryos—Blastocysts

To Be Prepared on the Day Before

- Prepare culture dishes containing eight 25 µL droplets of culture medium under oil and keep at 37°C.

Preparations on the Day (One to Two Hours before Thawing Cells)

- Take out collection and thawing media from the refrigerator (4°C) and equilibrate them at 22°C–26°C.

Procedure

- Identify the patients and straws for thawing and remove them from the liquid nitrogen containers into a dewar with liquid nitrogen.
- Thaw the straws by putting them first on the bench of a laminar air flow cabinet for 30 to 40 seconds at 22°C–26°C followed by shaking the straw in a 37°C warm water bath until all ice crystals have disappeared.
- After cutting the straw, empty the straw into thawing medium A and equilibrate for 5 min at 22°C–26°C.
- Pipette the cell(s) into thawing medium B and equilibrate for 5 min at 22°C–26°C.
- Pipette the cell(s) into collection medium and equilibrate for 5 min at 22°C–26°C (1).
- Pipette the cell(s) into collection medium and equilibrate for 5 min at 22°C–26°C (2).
- Warm the culture dish (2) with collection medium and the thawed cells to 37°C and equilibrate for 5 min.
- Pipette the cell(s) into a culture dish with 37°C warm culture medium.
- Evaluate the cell(s) for morphological survival under the microscope with heated stage.
- Put the culture dish containing the cell(s) in an incubator.

BIBLIOGRAPHY

Borini, A. et al. 2010. "Multicenter Observational Study on Slow Cooling Oocyte Cryopreservation: Clinical Outcome." *Fertility and Sterility* 94: 1662–8.

Edgar, D. and D. Gook. 2012. "A Critical Appraisal of Cryopreservation (Slow Cooling Versus Vitrification) of Human Oocytes and Embryos." *Human Reproduction Update* 18: 536–40.

Lassalle, B. et al. 1985. "Human Embryo Features that Influence the Success of Cryopreservation with the Use of 1,2-Propanediol." *Fertility and Sterility* 44: 645–51.

Mazur, P. 1990. "Equilibrium, Quasi Equilibrium and Non-Equilibrium Freezing of Mammalian Embryos." *Cell Biophysics* 17: 53–91.

Van den Abbeel, E. et al. 2005. "Slow Controlled Rate Freezing of Sequentially Cultured Human Blastocysts: An Evaluation of Two Freezing Strategies." *Human Reproduction* 20: 2939–45.

17

Oocyte Selection

Basak Balaban

Principles

- Selecting the most viable oocyte that would give rise to a healthy offspring is one of the most critical steps that controls the success rates in IVF/ICSI cycles.
- Morphology, despite being the most commonly used method in routine practice, is subjective, with limited predictive value, so there's a need for more objective criteria for oocyte selection.

Morphology

- Optimal oocyte morphology is defined as an oocyte with spherical structure enclosed by a uniform zona pellucida, with a uniform translucent cytoplasm free of inclusions and a size-appropriate polar body.
- Several morphological varieties of human metaphase-II (MII) oocytes have been characterized.
    - Cytoplasmic abnormalities:
        - Cytoplasmic granulations (slightly diffused or excessive whole/centrally located granulation) refractile bodies.
        - Smooth endoplasmic reticulum clusters (sERCs).
        - Vacuolization.
    - Extracytoplasmic abnormalities:
        - Dysmorphic zona pellucida.
        - Discoloration.
        - Shape anomalies.
        - Perivitelline space (PVS) appearance and debris in PVS.
        - First polar body morphology.
    - Gigantic sized oocytes; oocytes with gigantic first polar body.

Examination of Morphology

- MII oocyte morphology should be examined under an inverted microscope at a minimum of 200× magnification.

- The deviations that should be examined with high priority are in the following order:

    1. Gigantic-sized oocytes and oocytes that have a large first polar body.
    2. Presence of smooth endoplasmic reticulum cluster(s) within the cytoplasm.
    3. Presence of vacuole(s) within the cytoplasm (cut-off value 14 μm).
    4. Presence of organelle clustering/centrally located condensed granulation within the cytoplasm.
    5. Oocytes with refractile bodies/cytoplasmic inclusions or with dark cytoplasm/dark cytoplasm-granular cytoplasm/dark cytoplasm with slight granulation/dark granular appearance of the cytoplasm/diffused cytoplasmic granularity.
    6. Ovoid oocytes with ovoid zona and normally shaped oolemma, or ovoid zona and ovoid oolemma.
    7. Oocytes with extremely large perivitelline space (PVS).
    8. Dysmorphic zona pellucida, discoloration of the oocyte, first polar body morphology and debris in PVS.

Spindle Imaging

- Visualization of meiotic spindle (MS) presence and location in human MII oocytes by polarized microscopy has been examined as an objective tool for oocyte selection.
- However, MS formation and its deviations are not static phenomena but dynamic ones, that could be affected by physical and chemical procedures held in the embryology laboratory. Thus the relevance of such changes is still unclear and limited.
- Despite its prognostic value for IVF/ICSI clinical outcome, it might be scientifically inspiring to increase our knowledge of gametes and meiosis.

Practical Approaches to Assess Spindle by Polarized Microscopy

- The assessment of MS properties is performed under a polarized microscope, with specifically designed glass structured Petri dishes for a clear visualization.
- Even though the presence of first polar body is an objective sign of maturity of the oocyte, and the presence of MS is expected to be adjacent to it, the spindle presence might not be seen during the completion of the nuclear and cytoplasmic maturation period (mainly at the telophase I stage of development).
- Repetitive visualization checks within the 2–4 h of collection and denudation might be required after oocyte retrieval.
- The microtubules of the MS are highly sensitive to chemicals (hyaluronidase) and physical changes (temperature and pH variations) that may occur during oocyte handling.
- Shift of the PB1 position may also be related to physical displacement during denudation.
- Precise classification of spindle imaging should be performed repeatedly: after hyaluronidase treatment and immediately prior to ICSI.

Cumulus Gene Expression

- Cumulus cells are in close contact with the oocyte allowing an intense bi-directional communication between the two compartments during folliculogenesis and oocyte maturation.
- Gene expression profiling of the cumulus cells could be an important indicator and biomarker of oocyte quality.
- Even though multiple groups of genes expressed in follicular cells have been identified as possible indicators of oocyte maturity and viability, there is still a general lack of uniformity concerning groups of gene biomarkers among different studies.

Practical Approaches for Cumulus Cell Collection and Analysis

- Individual follicle aspiration is required for an objective analysis.
- Oocytes are injected and cultured individually.
- Cumulus cells are immediately removed from the oocytes by mechanical stripping using a needle and a glass denudation pipette.
- After being washed in preferably phosphate-buffered solution to remove blood cell contamination, they are snap frozen in liquid nitrogen and stored at −80°C until RNA isolation.

- RNA extraction should be performed by ready-to-use commercial kits.
- qRT-PCR is performed by gene expression pre-designed assays.

Follicular Fluid (FF) Assessment for Oocyte Selection

- Various components of follicular fluid are suggested as biochemical predictors of oocyte quality.
- Despite the lack of prospective validation, the majority of the clinical trials are performed on the detection of granulocyte colony-stimulating factor(G-CSF) quantified in individual FF of the representing oocyte.

Practical Approaches for Follicular Fluid Collection and Analysis

- Individual follicle aspiration is required for an objective analysis.
- Pooling of the samples is strongly discouraged.
- Oocytes are injected and cultured individually.
- Follicular fluid aspirated from each individual follicle should be collected separately and assayed if oocyte retrieval is successful.
- Recovered samples are centrifuged to remove debris and then divided in aliquots.
- Aliquots are stored initially at −20°C and then at −80°C until they are assayed for any hormone or protein of interest using commercially available ELISA kits (i.e., leptin) or non-ELISA micro-bead assay technology (i.e., G-CSF).

BIBLIOGRAPHY

Alpha Scientists in Reproductive Medicine and ESHRE Special Interest Group Embryology. 2011. "Istanbul Consensus Workshop on Embryo Assessment: Proceedings of an Expert Meeting." *Reproductive Biomedicine Online* 22: 632–46.

Fragouli, E., M.D. Lalioti, and D. Wells. 2014. "The Transcriptome of Follicular Cells: Biological Insights and Clinical Implications for the Treatment of Infertility." *Human Reproduction Update* 20: 1–11.

Ledee, N., V. Gridelet, S. Ravet, et al. 2013. "Impact of Follicular G-CSF Quantification on Subsequent Embryo Transfer Decisions: A Proof of Concept Study." *Human Reproduction* 28: 406–413.

Montag, M., M. Köster, K. Van der Ven, and H. Van der Ven. 2011. "Gamete Competence Assessment by Polarizing Optics in Assisted Reproduction." *Human Reproduction Update* 17: 654–66.

Rienzi, L., B. Balaban, T. Ebner, and J. Mandelbaum. 2012. "The Oocyte." *Human Reproduction* 27: i2–i21.

18

Zygote Selection

Martin Greuner

Principle

- Scoring of pronuclear characteristics, polar body positioning and a halo at the outer lining underneath the oolemma is used by some to assess the potential of a fertilized oocyte.

Required Equipment

- Sterile pipettes for stripping the remaining cumulus-coronal cells away 15–17 h after ICSI/IVF
- Inverted microscope with Hoffmann modulation differential contrast optics at magnifications of 400× and 600× with heated plate
- Photo-documentation

To Be Prepared on the Day Before

- Prepare the dishes for single-cell culture in droplets or wells.
- Equilibrate overnight in culture conditions (CO_2, reduced O_2 if applicable, 37°C).

Preparation on the Day

- Warm the heating plate of the microscope to 37°C.
- Prepare all equipment in the area of the working place to make sure that the cells are out of the incubator for as short a time as possible.
- Label all materials (scoring sheet and pipettes with patient identification items).

Zygote Selection

- Identify patient/materials for the patients.
- 15–17 h after IVF/ICSI strip the remaining cumulus-coronal cells away.
- Separate the cells in single culture in droplets or wells.
- Place the cells under the microscope 400×.

- Score the number of pronuclei.
- Documentation on the patient sheet.
- Locate the pronuclei (PN) in one plane (if not, turn the cells with the pipette until PN are aligned).
- Photo-document the cells with 600× and do a fast first scoring of all 2 PN.
- Place the dish back into the incubator.
- Verify the first scoring by comparing with the documented photos.
- Perform a detailed scoring based on the photo-documentation for the number of nucleolar precursor bodies (NPBs)/presence of a halo/polar body number and orientation.

Scoring of the Pronuclei

- Size of the pronuclei:
  - Equal or unequal.
- Position of the pronuclei:
  - Close together or well separated.
  - PN stage with two pronuclei that are not of the same size or that are not aligned at the center of the oocyte show a reduced development potential (Z4).
- Position, size and number of NPB:
  - Z1: Both pronuclei with equal numbers and size of NPB (nucleoli between three and seven) aligned or beginning to align at the pronuclear junction.
  - Z2: Both pronuclei with equal numbers and size of NPB which are equally scattered in the two pronuclei.
  - Z3: Both pronuclei with inequality of numbers and size or alignment of NPB.
  - Z4:
    - Both pronuclei of different size or not aligned in a center position in the cell.
    - NPB present as only one big NPB in one pronuclei (bull eye).
    - Pronuclei with no NPB (ghosts).

- The Z-scoring range is from Z1 (very good prognosis) to Z4 (bad prognosis).
- **Important:** Consider the timing of the scoring because the scores change in time and the NPB disappears before membrane breakdown.

Polar Body Positioning

- The positioning of the polar body can have a scoring character. The angle between the two polar bodies and the plane of the nearest polar body to the orientation of the pronuclei seem to have no influence, but the angle to the furthest polar body could relate to embryo quality—although this assumption has to be proven. Equally, the appearance of the polar body is in discussion.

Presence of the So-Called Halo

- Most of the zygotes display a halo but in a different specificity. It appears because of the transport from mitochondria towards the pronuclei. However, the importance and the meaning of symmetrical and polar halos are not yet understood. It could be that the halo appears and disappears and extreme or concentric halos could have a negative influence.

General

- After scoring, culture embryos individually to the desired transfer stage, take PN scoring into account together with morphology at the day of transfer.

BIBLIOGRAPHY

Alpha Scientists in Reproductive Medicine and ESHRE Special Interest Group Embryology. 2011. "Istanbul Consensus Workshop on Embryo Assessment: Proceedings of an Expert Meeting." *Reproductive Biomedicine Online* 22: 632–46.

Garello, C., H. Baker, J. Rai, S. Montgomery, P. Wilson, C.R. Kennedy, and G.M. Hartshorne. 1999. "Pronuclear Orientation, Polar Body Placement, and Embryo Quality After Intracytoplasmic Sperm Injection and in-Vitro Fertilization: Further Evidence for Polarity in Human Oocytes." *Human Reproduction* 14: 2588–95.

Greuner, M. and M. Montag. "Morphological Selection of Gametes and Embryos: 2PN/Zygote." *Selecting Gametes and Embryos*. Boca Raton, FL: CRC Press, 2014.

Scott, L. and S. Smith. 1998. "The Successful Use of Pronuclear Embryo Transfers the Day Following Oocyte Retrieval." *Human Reproduction* 13: 1003–13.

Scott, L., R. Alvero, M. Leondiris, and B. Miller. 2000. "The Morphology of Human Pronuclear Embryos Is Positively Related to Blastocyst Development and Implantation." *Human Reproduction* 15: 2394–403.

19

Selection and Grading of Embryos on Day 2/3 and Blastocysts on Day 5/6

Thorir Hardarson and Julius Hreinsson

Required Equipment

- Inverted microscope with heated plate and Hoffman modulation optics at 200× magnification
- Documentation chart and/or a digital registration system

Performing the Embryo Grading—General Points

- Work as quickly as possible to minimize exposure to ambient air.
- Ideally, two embryologists perform the grading together, one working the microscope and manipulating embryos, the other registering the observations, both contributing to the decision-making process.
- The embryo grading parameters are based on the ESHRE/Alpha consensus document.

Early Cleavage

- Early cleavage check is performed 26 ± 1 hr post ICSI and 28 ± 1 h post IVF insemination.
- Oocytes in syngamy (PN disappeared) and early cleaved oocytes (2 cells) are documented.
- Optimal embryos are at the 2-cell stage at this time.
- Oocytes in syngamy are considered normal.
- Oocytes displaying 2PN at this time have reduced speed of development.
- Embryos having cleaved into three or more cells have severely reduced developmental potential. This is, however, often difficult to assess with certainty unless time-lapse equipment is used.

Grading Parameters on Day 2/3

- Recommended times for assessment are 44 ± 1 h post-insemination (day 2) and 68 ± 1 h post-insemination (day 3).
- The optimal day 2 embryo has four equally sized mononucleated cells in a tetrahedral arrangement with <10% fragmentation.
- The optimal day 3 embryo has eight equally sized mononucleated cells with <10% fragmentation.
- Developmental potential is slightly reduced for 5–6 cell embryos on day 2 and severely reduced for 2–3 or 7–8 cell embryos on day 2.
- Developmental potential is slightly reduced for 6–7 cell embryos or 9–12 cell embryos on day 3 and severely reduced for <6 cell embryos and >12 cell embryos on day 3.
- Developmental potential is reduced with increasing degrees of fragmentation where more than 25% fragmentation is associated with severe reduction.
- Binucleate cells may be observed at earlier stages of development (2–4 cells) and may be a sign of reduced potential. Multinucleated cells are considered beyond repair and increasing numbers of these cells in the embryo will severely reduce its potential.
- Cell size should be stage-specific where 2, 4 and 8 cell embryos should have equally sized cells. Large deviations (>25%) from expected cell size correlate with reduced developmental potential.
- Other parameters, such as cytoplasmic granularity and zona pellucida anomalies such as shape deformation, have a more unclear association with embryo developmental potential but are usually considered negative prognostic factors.

Grading Parameters on Day 5/6

- The recommended time for assessment is 116±2 h post insemination on day 5.
- The optimal blastocyst is at this time expanded or hatching with a prominent inner cell mass (ICM) and a trophectoderm (TE) containing many cells, forming a cohesive epithelium. Both ICM and TE are important for further development.
- As blastocyst development is delayed from the 116 h, developmental potential is reduced where fully developed blastocysts on day 5 are considered having greatest potential. Viable blastocysts can be identified on day 6 or even on day 7 post insemination, but for practical reasons, blastocysts are usually not cultured after day 6.
- ICM is scored as having good quality when the cells are numerous, prominent and compacted; average quality where cells are loosely grouped together; and poor quality when the ICM contains few cells and is difficult to discern.
- TE is scored as having good quality when containing numerous cells forming a cohesive epithelium; average quality when containing few cells and loose epithelium; poor quality when containing few cells.
- The potential effect of anomalies such as cytoplasmic strings is unclear, but incomplete cavitation is considered a negative prognostic factor.

Additional Parameters for Time-Lapse Monitoring

- Continuous monitoring of embryo development using time-lapse technology has greatly increased our understanding of the dynamics of embryo development. This technology, as currently used, allows visualization of embryo development in intervals as small as 10 minutes, while simultaneously allowing uninterrupted culture.
- The most important parameters added to the scheme above are visualization of irregular cleavage patterns, for example when a cell produces three daughter cells. The earlier this occurs in development, the greater the negative prognostic effect. Also, the timing of cell cycles and synchronicity of cleavage can be observed. For example, in a 2-cell embryo, each cell should cleave to two daughter cells with very short time intervals between the two. That is to say, the 3-cell stage of embryo development should be very short, or preferably non-existent. Also, the timing of PN appearance (from 6–8 h post insemination) and disappearance (approximately 20 h post insemination) can be observed and any deviations can be noted.

- It should be noted that the use of time-lapse in IVF is still in its infancy and, although it shows much promise, it still needs further study to be able to be used as a predictor of a viable pregnancy. In addition, there are several cell cleavage patterns that at present are difficult to assess, as the cellular cleavages are sometimes incomplete and move back and forward in number.

Decision Making and Weight of Parameters

- External factors such as stress, fatigue and visual or other disturbances will affect decision making negatively. Having two embryologists evaluating embryo development simultaneously as mentioned above will improve the process.
- Weighing the scoring parameters is not unequivocal and there is no international consensus for this important task, even though a majority of patients have more than one cleaving embryo to select for transfer and/or cryopreservation. It is crucial to apply single embryo transfer as much as possible, or at least to >75% of cases, since transferring multiple embryos will mostly only increase multiple pregnancy rates and not significantly increase pregnancy rates per patient.

How to Interpret Systematic Anomalies in Embryo Grading

- Abnormally high levels of multinucleated embryos (>30%) may indicate anomalies in the temperature control chain in the laboratory.
- Slow development or lack of blastocyst development may indicate a toxic effect in the culture system.

BIBLIOGRAPHY

Alpha Scientists in Reproductive Medicine and ESHRE Special Interest Group of Embryology. 2011. "The Istanbul Consensus Workshop on Embryo Assessment: Proceedings of an Expert Meeting." *Human Reproduction* 26(6): 1270–83.

Flin, R., P. O'Connor, and M. Crichton. *Safety at the Sharp End: A Guide to Non-Technical Skills.* Ashgate Publishing Ltd., 2008.

Rubio, I., A. Galán, Z. Larreategui, F. Ayerdi, J. Bellver, J. Herrero, and M. Meseguer. 2014. "Clinical Validation of Embryo Culture and Selection by Morphokinetic Analysis: A Randomized, Controlled Trial of the EmbryoScope." *Fertility and Sterility* 102(5): 1287–94.

20

Time-Lapse Imaging

Cristina Hickman

Required Equipment

- Time-lapse incubator
- Time-lapse incubator dish
- Single-step bicarbonate buffered media with protein supplementation
- Oil for overlay
- Software to annotate videos
- Statistical software to analyze morphokinetic data
- Pipettors (135 μm, 200 μm)
- Multipette dispenser and 1 mL CombiTips
- Handheld CO_2 monitor
- Handheld temperature monitor
- Handheld blood gas analyzer

Installation and Validation

- Place time-lapse incubator on a stable bench in an area with clean, VOC-free grade C (or above) air and stable temperature control with access to medical grade nitrogen and carbon dioxide gases, 24/7 alarm system and an in-line UPS. Plugs should be resistant to being pulled out.
- Set up a quality management system around time lapse, including SOP of how to maintain, monitor and use the equipment, annotation definitions, competency assessment of how to annotate, quality control of annotations (to identify errors and blanks), and frequent validation of method for selection of embryos (the frequency will vary according to the number of cycles cultured in time-lapse).
- As a guide, every 3–6 months (if performing 500 cycles), validate embryo selection data with regards to sensitivity and specificity of predicting implantation potential.
- Set up a process for patients to receive videos (either using USBs or an option to download videos online).

Day before Egg Collection

- Bring the media to room temperature. Avoid evaporation by not preparing dishes on a heated stage, and reduce bubble formation by not using media straight from the fridge.
- Prepare a maximum of two dishes at a time to avoid evaporation.
- Using the 145 μm pipettor (or smaller) under a stereo microscope at around 10× magnification, add about 2 μL of media into the inside of each of the inner wells of the time-lapse dish.
- Using multipette, aliquot 23 μL into each of the 12 embryo culture wells and the four wash wells.
- Immediately overlay with oil.
- Incubate time-lapse dishes overnight (around 16 hours) at $37 \pm 1°C$, 5%–7.5% carbon dioxide (depending on media pH validation), 5%–6% oxygen.

On the Day of Egg Collection

- In the morning, remove any air bubbles in the time-lapse dishes using a 145 μL pipettor and return the time-lapse dishes to the incubator as quickly as possible (within four minutes).
- Time-lapse allows for insemination to occur without the time restrictions for pronucleate checking. Therefore, short gamete co-incubation may be adopted. If conventional IVF is to be performed, expose COCs destined for IVF to sperm not before 1 hour from the end of egg collection. Gamete co-incubation occurs for a minimum of 2 hours, preferably between 4 and 6 hours. At the end of gamete co-incubation, oocytes are stripped if the cumulus appears dispersed (in cases of undispersed cumulus, gamete co-incubation is extended to overnight only for the affected oocytes). Oocytes with dispersed cumulus are only partially stripped before assessment of maturity. Immature oocytes are returned to the dish containing sperm and cultured

overnight, while mature oocytes are washed thoroughly from sperm and debris and placed in the time-lapse dish. The amount of sperm and debris from the co-incubation dish transferred to the time-lapse dish should be avoided and monitored per practitioner.

- Wash oocytes thoroughly using the four wash wells of the dish and then place oocytes in minimum volume in the center of the inner well.
- Place the dish inside the time-lapse incubator and push the dish down onto the dish holder.
- Record the time of end of ICSI or the time of IVF sperm exposure (as applicable) as the time of insemination.
- Check the images are all in focus.

What Steps to Take in the Procedure Itself

- From days 0 to 6, annotate the embryological events using the definitions outlined in the SOP. In case a time-lapse-based embryo selection model is in place, only the embryological events included in the embryo selection model need to be annotated. Annotations may take place at any time before embryo transfer, although the bulk of annotations should be performed on days preceding embryo transfer day.
- Preferably, culture embryos to day 5 or 6 after egg collection (this will maximize number of parameters collected). Select embryos based on the following criteria:
  - Give preference to embryos [double pronuclei (2PN) or single (1PN)] that form a blastocyst.
  - De-select embryos that direct cleaved from 1 to 3 cells in the first cell division (cells and fragments can be differentiated by observation of a nucleus, further cell divisions, and/or inclusion in the morula formation).
  - De-select embryos that divided to 2 cells beyond 32 hours.
  - De-select embryos with multinucleation observed in all cells at the 4-cell stage.
  - Give preference to embryos with better trophectoderm morphology and visible inner cell mass.
  - Give preference to embryos with the highest score using multiple validated models. Some devices have software that automatically score and rank the embryos according to morphokinetic parameters.
  - Give preference to embryos that have tSB less than 110 hpi, and have reached the most expanded stage according to Gardner grading.
  - De-select embryos with 1PN, uneven and/or separate pronuclei, asynchronous pronuclear appearance and disappearance.
  - Give preference to embryos with increased evenness and less fragmentation at the 4-cell stage.
- Extract a video of the embryos selected for transfer onto a USB stick.
- Extract a report with pictures of the embryos suitable for cryopreservation onto a USB stick.
- Explain the embryological observations to the patient using the video and the picture report.
- Extrapolate chances of pregnancy based on age and observations.

Model Building and Validation Using Statistics Software

- Add the clinical outcome to the dataset and ensure the completeness of the dataset, particularly with regard to interrupted videos, missed annotations, and missed outcomes (implantation or live birth). Perform all operations on an export of the time-lapse variables in a database (such as Microsoft Excel). Statistics can be performed using a statistics software package.
- Models can be built on parameters for variables from embryos with known implantation data (KID), provided that the data quality is high (correct annotation; no missing values; outcome data available).
- Classify the embryos into KID positive (embryos were transferred and the number of gestational sacs or fetal heartbeats equals the number of transferred embryos), KID negative (embryos that were transferred and did not implant) and KID unknown (embryos were transferred and the number of gestational sacs or fetal heartbeats is less than the number of transferred embryos). Only KID positive or KID negative embryos may be used to calculate KID ratio (KID positive/KID negative).
- Calculate the KID ratio for each morphokinetic parameter window. Consider also using time intervals between absolute variables (i.e., cc2, cc3). Deselection parameters will have a low KID ratio, while selection parameters will have a high KID ratio. Rank the various selection and deselection parameters according to diagnostic odds ratio (DOR). Build in morphological assessments into the same ranking and prioritize decision making according to highest DOR. Statistical software may be used to calculate Area Under the Curve to further assist model building and embryo selection decision making. Models should be reviewed using new data every 3–6 months. In particular, cycles where fresh transfer lead to no pregnancy but subsequent frozen transfers from the same original fresh cycles lead to a pregnancy may be used to further validate the proposed models before implementation.

BIBLIOGRAPHY

Ciray, H.N., A. Campbell, I.E. Agerholm, J. Aguilar, S. Chamayou, M. Esbert, S. Sayed, Time-Lapse User Group. 2014. "Proposed Guidelines on the Nomenclature and Annotation of Dynamic Human Embryo Monitoring by a Time-Lapse User Group." *Human Reproduction* 29(12): 2650–60.

21

Assisted Hatching

Christian De Geyter and Maria De Geyter

Principles

- Observational studies have demonstrated that failure of embryos to implant may result from their inability to escape the zona pellucida.
- Hardening of the zona pellucida during embryo culture has been made responsible for failed embryo hatching, or increased zona thickness as caused by female infertility.
- Artificial opening of the zona pellucida, so-called assisted hatching or thinning of the zona pellucida, has been proposed to overcome this problem.
- Early studies have demonstrated beneficial effects of assisted hatching in poor-prognosis embryos with thickened zona pellucida.

Required Equipment

- Although various methods, including mechanical hatching, have been proposed, two methods are currently widely used: thinning of the zona pellucida with acidic Tyrode's solution or with a laser beam.
- For the purpose of opening the zona pellucida with a 1.48 µm diode laser beam, an inverted microscope needs to be equipped with a heated plate, with a micromanipulator (only for using acidic Tyrode's solution) and with a laser system. The laser beam is then directed by several mirrors through a 40× objective (compatible with the laser wavelength) of the inverted microscope towards the zona pellucida of the embryo to be treated.

Procedures

Assisted Hatching with Tyrode's Solution

See Chapter 22.

Assisted Hatching with a Laser Beam

- Preferably all embryos should be hatched on day 2, as at that stage of embryonic development the perivitelline space is the largest.
- The embryos are positioned in small 10 µL droplets of IVF-culture medium under paraffin oil.
- Place the dish with the embryos to be hatched on the heated place of an inverted microscope.
- Use the laser objective.
- Place the embryo so that the on-screen crosshair position that denotes the laser focus point does not target any portion of the cytoplasm of the oocyte.
- Target the crosshair position such that only the zona pellucida is targeted.
- Unlock the laser and set the laser beam to a pulse length that allows for the complete opening of the zona pellucida.
- **Note:** The pulse length required for a specific opening is dependent on several parameters like power of the laser diode, optical system (quality of lenses), distance between bottom of the dish to the target point in medium, and others. Therefore a specific pulse length in msec cannot be advised, but has to be defined for each individual setup.
- The size of the hole in the zona pellucida is to approximate the thickness of the zona pellucida.
- A second pulse may be needed to hatch all the way through the zona pellucida.
- Use the side button on the mouse to trigger the laser or any specific trigger device.
- If transfer of embryos is scheduled at the blastocyst stage, early hatching should be avoided because of the risk of premature hatching. Transfer of prematurely hatching of blastocyst embryos raises the risk of monozygotic twin pregnancy.
- Return the dish with the treated embryos to the incubator.

Effect of Assisted Hatching
on Treatment Outcome

- Only few prospective comparative (not randomized) studies were performed to compare the efficacy of different methods of assisted hatching. The outcome data of both methods including the clinical pregnancy rate seem to be similar.

- A systematic review of outcome studies has reported in 2012 that assisted hatching significantly contributes to improve the likelihood of achieving a clinical pregnancy. However, data on the impact of assisted hatching on live birth rates are insufficient to draw any conclusion.

BIBLIOGRAPHY

Balaban, B., B. Urman, C. Alatas, R. Mercan, et al. 2002. "A Comparison of Four Different Techniques of Assisted Hatching." *Human Reproduction* 17: 1239–43.

Carney, S.K., S. Das, D. Blake, C. Farquhar, et al. 2012. "Assisted Hatching on Assisted Conception (in Vitro Fertilisation (IVF) and Intracytoplasmic Sperm Injection (ICSI)." *Cochrane Database of Systematic Reviews* 12: CD001894.

Cohen, J., M. Alikani, J. Trowbridge, and Z. Rosenwaks. 1992. "Implantation Enhancement by Selective Assisted Hatching Using Zona Drilling of Human Embryos with Poor Prognosis." *Human Reproduction* 7: 685–91.

Schiewe, M.C., J.B. Whitney, and R.E. Anderson. 2015. "Potential Risk of Monochorionic Dizygotic Twin Blastocyst Formation Associated with Early Laser Zona Dissection of Group Cultured Embryos." *Fertility and Sterility* 103: 417–21.

Selva, J. 2000. "Assisted Hatching." *Human Reproduction* 15 (Suppl 4): 65–7.

22

Zona Manipulation at Various Embryo Stages: Mechanical/Acidic Medium

Marius Meintjes

Required Equipment

- Micromanipulator-equipped inverted microscope for zona manipulation (ZM) with 400× magnification capability
- Heated microscope stage at 36.5°C–37.0°C
- Holding pipette (100 mm OD; 30 mm ID)
- Assisted hatching pipette (10 mm OD) for chemical ZM
- Acid Tyrode's solution (pH approx. 2.5) (Sigma Aldrich, EMD Millipore) or acidified HTF (pH 2.4) (Origio)
- Partial zona dissection (PZD) needle for mechanical ZM
- Laminar flow hood for preparing manipulation and culture dishes
- Pipetting supplies to move embryos
- Gloves (non-powder) (*optional*)

To Be Prepared on the Day Before

- Confirm that appropriate consents and orders are in place to perform ZM.
- Confirm that all micromanipulation tools are in stock.
- Prepare 20 μL micro-drops under oil for each embryo in a micromanipulation dish using protein-, amino acid-supplemented and environmental-buffered (HEPES or MOPS) medium.
- Prepare enough dishes to accommodate all embryos.
- Prepare and equilibrate post-manipulation wash and culture dish overnight.
- Prepare an additional 20 μL micro-drop of acidified medium under oil in the same micromanipulation dish and circle/identify clearly.

Preparation on the Day

- Pre-warm the micromanipulation dish to 36.5°C–37.0°C.
- Ensure that the manipulation syringes, lines and tool holders are intact with the proper seals.
- Fit the microtools into the tool holders (typically, holding pipette on left and needle/pipette on right).
- Center the tools using coarse and fine adjustments.
- Check all fittings for tightness.
- Confirm patient identification and compliance with written orders/consent.

Zona Manipulation

Intended Use

- Assisted hatching of transfer-embryos for clinic-specified patient groups
- Assisted hatching of frozen-thawed blastocysts
- Zona breaching for day 3 biopsy of blastomeres
- Zona breaching in preparation for later trophectoderm biopsy
- Providing access for fragment removal

Mechanical

- Place one to three embryos in each 20 μL micromanipulation droplet.
- Using the holding pipette, position and secure cleavage-stage embryos to present with the largest possible perivitelline space towards the tip of the PZD needle.
- Blastocyst contraction can first be induced by pricking the trophoblast with the PZD needle through the zona pellucida (ZP). The blastocyst can then be orientated with the ICM away from the manipulation area.

- Penetrate the ZP approximately at the 2 o'clock position.
- Then, slant the needle towards 12 o'clock and exit the ZP approximately at the 10 o'clock position, but still above the holding pipette.
- Refrain from damaging blastomeres or trophoblast cells during this process.
- Release the hold of the holding pipette.
- Rub the trapped ZP area against the holding pipette in carefully executed saw-like motions until the PZD needle has traversed this span of zona between the 10 o'clock and 2 o'clock penetrations, leaving a linear 40–50 μm cut.
- When performing a simultaneous biopsy or fragment removal procedure, a double tool holder can be used.
- Alternatively, exchange for a biopsy- or fragment removal tool and rotate the embryos with the ZP defect towards the biopsy/fragment-removal pipette.
- After completion of the procedure, rinse embryos in culture medium and then transfer to the culture dish for continued culture in 5.5%–6.5% CO_2/5% O_2.

Chemical

- Place one embryo only in each 20 μL micromanipulation droplet.
- Make sure to wash the embryos as soon as possible after drilling and do not use drops twice. This is important to protect the embryos from prolonged exposure to a possible lowered medium pH that can result from using the low-pH drilling fluid in a small culture medium volume.
- Preload the drilling pipette with acid Tyrode's or acidified HTF, ensuring a working intra-pipette pH of approximately 2.5.
- Allow the drilling pipette to fill halfway between the tip and the area of widest pipette diameter.
- Elevate the pipette tip from and above the acidified medium micro droplet.
- Position and secure cleavage-stage embryos to present with a large perivitelline space or fragments towards the drilling pipette.
- Induced blastocyst contraction is not required, but always position the ICM away from the area of ZM.
- Lower the prefilled drilling pipette into the ZM droplet while applying slight positive pressure. This will prevent capillary action-mediated dilution of the drilling acid by holding-drop medium.
- Now apply micro-pulses of acidic medium directly onto the ZP, maintaining close proximity to the embryo.
- While pulsing, move the 10–12 μm diameter pipette gently up and down to evenly expose the ZP to undiluted acid over a longitudinal 25–30 μm area.

- After the ZP has been thinned sufficiently over this 25–30 μm area, concentrate the pulses of acidic medium in a small localized zone towards the center of this working area.
- The concentrated pulses should eventually result in a bulging film-like behavior of the now significantly thinned ZP.
- When this bulging is observed, finally penetrate the ZP by applying slight suction rather than by continuing to blow through the ZP. When blowing through instead of penetrating the ZP with suction, surplus acidic medium may end up in the perivitelline space, which is not desirable.
- After penetration of the ZP, again maintain slight positive pressure to prevent dilution of the acidic medium inside the pipette, ensuring continued drilling efficiency for the next embryo.
- Lift the drilling pipette from the ZM droplet.
- If at any time ZP dissolving efficiency is lost, reprime the pipette with fresh acidic solution.
- After successful drilling of each embryo, move the embryo around in the manipulation droplet with the holding pipette to relieve any acid accumulation around the embryo.
- For subsequent biopsy, a double tool holder can be used with the appropriate biopsy pipette.
- Alternatively, exchange the drilling pipette for a biopsy pipette and then carefully rotate the embryo so that the ZP defect faces the biopsy pipette.
- For fragment removal, the acid solution can be expelled in an empty medium droplet and then the same pipette can be used for fragment removal, without having to change pipettes or the need for a double tool holder.
- Rinse embryos in culture medium and then transfer to the culture dish for continued culture in 5.5–6.5% CO_2/5% O_2.

Laser

- Refer to Chapter 21 for details on laser zona manipulation.

BIBLIOGRAPHY

Balaban, B., B. Urman, C. Alatas, R. Mercan, A. Mumcu, and A. Isiklar. 2002. "A Comparison of Four Different Techniques of Assisted Hatching." *Human Reproduction* 17(5): 1239–43.

Baruffi, R., A. Mauri, C. Petersen, R. Ferreira, J. Coelho, and J. Franco. 2000. "Zona Thinning with Noncontact Diode Laser in Patients Aged <37 Years with No Previous Failure of Implantation: A Prospective Randomized Study." *Journal of Assisted Reproduction and Genetics* 17: 557–60.

Cieslak, J., V. Ivakhnenko, G. Wolf, S. Shelag, and Y. Verlinsky. 1999. "Three-Dimensional Partial Zona Dissection for Preimplantation Genetic Diagnosis and Assisted Hatching." *Fertility and Sterility* 71: 308–13.

Cohen, J., M. Alikani, J. Trowbridge, and Z. Rozenwaks. 1992. "Implantation Enhancement by Selective Assisted Hatching Using Zona Drilling of Embryos with Poor Prognosis." *Human Reproduction* 7: 685–91.

Jones, A., G. Wright, H. Kort, R. Straub, and Z. Nagy. 2006. "Comparison of Laser-Assisted Hatching and Acidified Tyrode's Hatching by Evaluation of Blastocyst Development Rates in Sibling Embryos: A Prospective Randomized Trial." *Fertility and Sterility* 85(2): 487–91.

23

Biopsy: Polar Body, Blastomere, Trophectoderm

Hakan Yelke and Semra Kahraman

Required Equipment

- Stereo microscope with heated plate
- Laminar flow hood with built-in heated plate
- Heating plate/warm incubator
- Inverted microscope with heated stage (37°C), laser and micromanipulators

Required Consumables

- ICSI dish
- Ca^{2+}/Mg^{2+} free HEPES-buffered culture medium for blastomere biopsy (BB)
- HEPES-buffered culture medium (containing Ca^{2+}/Mg^{2+}) for polar body biopsy (PBB) and trophectoderm biopsy (TB)
- Sterile light paraffin oil
- PBB (ID: 18–21 μm) or BB pipette (30–35 μm) BB pipette used also for TB
- Holding pipette
- Mouth controlled holder for TB
- Stripper and tips (150–155 μm for PBB; 150–250 μm for BB and TB)
- PBS (phosphate-buffered saline) solution

Preparation on the Biopsy Day

- Pre-warm all heating devices to the appropriate temperature.
- Prepare the biopsy dish at least 20 min before the manipulation and warm it to 37°C.
- Prepare 3 columns and 4 rows of 9 μL drops with:
  - Ca^{2+}/Mg^{2+} free HEPES-buffered culture medium for BB.
  - HEPES-buffered culture medium (containing Ca^{2+}/Mg^{2+}) for PBB or TB.
- Cover the droplets with 4 mL pre-warmed sterile light paraffin oil (37°C).

- Mark the name of the patient and the number of MII oocytes/cleavage-stage embryos/blastocysts to be biopsied on the bottom of the biopsy dish.

Zona Opening Procedure by Laser

Polar Body Biopsy

Perform PBB post-fertilization (8–9 h post-ICSI) to remove both the first and the second PB simultaneously. At that time frame, PB1 is free in the perivitelline space but PB2 is slightly connected to the oolemma with a cytoplasmic strand. [*Optional:* Consecutive PBB can be performed: 4 h post-ICSI PB1 and >8 h post-ICSI PB2.]

- Care should be taken to denude completely MII oocytes to be biopsied to avoid contamination by cumulus cells.
- Take the previously prepared and pre-warmed biopsy dish.
- Transfer MII oocytes into the first column of droplets containing HEPES-buffered culture medium.
- Wash several times to remove any residual culture medium.
- Hold and position the MII oocyte with a holding pipette.
- Create an opening of 10–15 μm in diameter on the ZP by laser or mechanical.
- Make sure that PB1, PB2 and the opening in the ZP are at the same focal plane as the biopsy pipette.
- Introduce the PB pipette through the opening created on the ZP.
- Apply gentle suction to remove PB1 and put it at the 12 o'clock position in the same drop without releasing the MII oocyte.
- Introduce the PB pipette again through the opening created on the ZP.
- Apply gentle suction to remove PB2 and put it at the 6 o'clock position in the same drop.
- Release the MII oocyte from the holding pipette.

- Place the biopsy dish on the heated stage of the laminar flow hood.
- Take out the biopsied MII oocyte from the biopsy medium.
- Place it into the dish with routine culture medium after several washings to remove any residual HEPES-buffered medium (check patient name or label now).
- Place the dish back into the gassed incubator.

Blastomere Biopsy

BB is mostly performed on embryos with at least 7 blastomeres on day 3, which corresponds to 65–72 hours after insemination.

- Assess the morphology of the embryo(s) to be biopsied.
- Take the previously prepared and pre-warmed biopsy dish.
- Transfer embryos into the first column of droplets containing Ca^{2+}/Mg^{2+} free HEPES-buffered culture medium.
- Wash several times to remove any residual culture medium and move them in the second column, same row.
- Wait for 2–3 minutes in order to reversibly loosen the membrane adhesion between blastomeres.
- Care should be taken to minimize the time of manipulation during the biopsy procedure.
- After the incubation, evaluate the blastomere to be biopsied for the presence of a proper nucleus and cytoplasmic appearance on the inverted microscope.
- Hold and position the embryo with a holding pipette.
- Create an opening of 10–20 μm in diameter on the ZP by laser or chemical or mechanical.
- Make sure that the blastomere to be biopsied, the opening in the ZP and the biopsy pipette are on the same focal plane.
- Introduce the BB pipette through the opening created on the ZP.
- Apply gentle suction to remove a single blastomere from the embryo.
- Release the embryo from the holding pipette.
- Put the aspirated blastomere in the droplet on the right of the biopsy droplet.
- Check for the presence of a nucleus.
- Place the biopsy dish on the heated stage of the laminar flow hood.
- Take out the biopsied embryo from the biopsy medium.
- Place it into the dish with routine culture medium after several washings to remove any residual Ca^{2+}/Mg^{2+} free medium (check patient name or label now).
- Place the dish back into the gassed incubator.

Trophectoderm Biopsy

TB is performed to blastocysts with trophectoderm (TE) cells herniating through the opening made in the ZP on day 3 or 4 (refer to Chapters 21 and 22).

- Assess the morphology of the blastocyst(s) to be biopsied.
- Take the previously prepared and pre-warmed biopsy dish.
- Transfer blastocysts into the first column of droplets containing HEPES-buffered culture medium.
- Wash several times to remove any residual culture medium and move the blastocysts into the second column, same row.
- Care should be taken to minimize the time of manipulation during the biopsy procedure.
- Position the blastocyst and hold with the capillary at the side opposite to the herniating TE cells to avoid any direct contact/damage to the herniating cells.
- Make sure that the piece to be biopsied, the opening in the ZP and the biopsy pipette are on the same plane.
- Smoothly aspirate the herniated TE cells (range 2 to 9 cells) with the BB pipette.
- Apply gentle suction pressure 1–2 time(s) to cause collapse of the herniated TE cells.
- Continue with a mechanical rubbing on the holding pipette to promote separation. [*Optional:* Use a combination of single laser pulses at TE cell junctions with mechanical stretching to separate the TE piece.]
- Release the blastocyst from the holding pipette.
- Put the aspirated TE cells in the droplet on the right of the biopsy droplet.
- Place the biopsy dish on the heated stage of the laminar flow hood.
- Take out the biopsied blastocyst from the biopsy medium.
- Place it into the dish with routine culture media after several washings to remove any residual HEPES-buffered medium (check patient name or label now).
- Place the dish back into the gassed incubator.

Transfer of Biopsied Material

- For aCGH, place the biopsied cells with a Stripper tip of 50 μm in diameter in a PCR tube filled with 2 μL PBS medium.
- A maximum volume of 0.5 μL of the biopsied sample can be carried to obtain a final volume of 2.5 μL.
- See also Chapter 24.

BIBLIOGRAPHY

de Boer, K.A., J.W. Catt, R.P. Jansen, D. Leigh, and S. McArthur. 2004. "Moving to Blastocyst Biopsy for Preimplantation Genetic Diagnosis and Single Embryo Transfer at Sydney IVF." *Fertility and Sterility* 82(2): 295–8.

Montag, M., N. Limbach, M. Sabarstinski, K. van der Ven, C. Dorn, and H. van der Ven. 2005. "Polar Body Biopsy and Aneuploidy Testing by Simultaneous Detection of Six Chromosomes." *Prenatal Diagnosis* 25(10): 867–71.

Munné, S., A. Lee, Z. Rosenwaks, J. Grifo, and J. Cohen. 1993. "Diagnosis of Major Chromosome Aneuploidies in Human Preimplantation Embryos." *Human Reproduction* 8(12): 2185–91.

24

Sampling of Cells after Biopsy for aCGH

Barry Behr

Cell Types

- Polar bodies
- Blastomeres
- Trophectoderm

Required Equipment

- Laminar flow hood
- Stereo microscope
- Sterile powder-free gloves
- Hat and mask
- Sterile PCR tubes and rack
- Indelible marker
- Sterile Petri dishes
- Pipetting device (i.e., Stripper) plus suitable tips
- Specimen collection kit (array wash buffer)
- Refrigerator/freezer
- Dry ice/ice packs

Precautions

- Never touch shipping tubes without gloves.
- Wear fresh gloves and face mask throughout the procedure.
- Change gloves if they accidentally make contact with a source of contamination, such as human skin.
- Use new Stripper tip for each specimen.
- Never open any PCR tubes, collection kit or array wash buffer (AWB) outside of a hood.

Sample Preparation and Loading

- Place the specimen collection kit containing the PCR collection tubes in the laminar hood.

- Sample preparation should be performed in a laminar flow hood using powder-free gloves to prevent possible DNA contamination.
- Take the AWB out of the refrigerator and place it in the laminar hood.
- Washing step is critical to avoid any sperm or cumulus cell contamination.
- Prior to performing biopsy, pipette four 15–20 μL drops of AWB onto a sterile dish.
- Label the collection tube(s) with the embryo number on both the cap and the side of the tube.
- Before removing the sample from the embryo biopsy dish, rinse the Stripper tip with 3 μL of fresh AWB by filling and then expelling two times.
- Using the same rinsed Stripper tip, transfer the sample to the first washing drop.
- Flush 3–5 μL of array washing buffer over the samples in order to move and roll it into a different area of the same drop. It is important to minimize the amount of fluid transferred from one wash drop to the next one.
- After the last washing step, add the biopsied cell(s) to the sterile collection tube. Ensure that the tube number that the cell(s) is being added to matches the correct biopsied embryo number. Transfer minimal amount of buffer with cells.
- Place the tubes into the rack. Place the lid onto the rack and seal the rack with a piece of laboratory tape.
- Label the box with the patient name and date of birth (or affix the patient label).

Shipping Specimens to the PGD Company

Note: Be sure to follow the specific shipping and packing instructions for the particular PGD company being used.

- Once all the samples have been collected in tubes and placed in the rack, put the clear plastic top on the rack. Tape all the side of the rack to ensure that it will not open during the shipment. Avoid flipping tubes or the rack.

- Use an insulated shipping box that is usually provided by the PGD company (styrofoam container in a cardboard box). Place the rack containing the PCR collection tubes in the styrofoam container, add dry ice and seal the shipping box.
- Include the biopsy worksheet, requisition, consents and any other required paperwork in the shipping box before sealing the box with shipping tape.

BIBLIOGRAPHY

Gutiérrez-Mateo, C., P. Colls, J. Sánchez-García, T. Escudero, R. Prates, K. Ketterson, D. Wells, and S. Munné. 2011. "Validation of Microarray Comparative Genomic Hybridization for Comprehensive Chromosome Analysis of Embryos." *Fertility and Sterility* 95(3): 953–8.

Johnson, D.S., G. Gemelos, J. Baner, A. Ryan, C. Cinnioglu, M. Banjevic, R. Ross, M. Alper, B. Barrett, J. Frederick, D. Potter, B. Behr, and M. Rabinowitz. 2010. "Preclinical Validation of a Microarray Method for Full Molecular Karyotyping of Blastomeres in a 24-H Protocol." *Human Reproduction* 25(4): 1066–75.

Yang, Z., J. Liu, G.S. Collins, S.A. Salem, X. Liu, S.S. Lyle, A.C. Peck, E.S. Sills, and R.D. Salem. 2012. "Selection of Single Blastocysts for Fresh Transfer Via Standard Morphology Assessment Alone and with Array CGH for Good Prognosis IVF Patients: Results From a Randomized Pilot Study." *Molecular Cytogenetics* 5(1): 24.

25

Embryo Transfer—Standard and Ultrasound Guided

Bettina Toth

Principles

- There are different techniques which are used in embryo transfer (ET). However, ET is one of several relevant factors affecting the success of assisted reproduction (ART).
- Physicians have to be aware that, beside the amount of culture medium (transferred together with the embryo), the presence of blood at the catheter tip or a large amount of mucus within the cervix as well as malformations or strictures within the cervix/uterine cavity and finally their own experience all have an impact on the outcome of ART.

Required Equipment

- Center-well dish for embryo transfer
- Embryo transfer culture medium
- Handling pipettes
- Embryo transfer catheter
- Specula
- Gauze pad
- Sterile water (e.g., sterile NaCl, no disinfectant)
- Pincer
- Ultrasound with 8–5 MHz vaginal and/or 5–2 MHz abdominal transducers
- Embryo transfer catheter (soft, echogenic)
- Gloves (non-powder)
- Documentation chart

To Be Prepared at Oocyte Pick-Up/ On the Day before Transfer

- Information of the patient and the team of the time and place of the embryo transfer.
- Mock transfer in case of malformations or strictures within the cervix/uterine cavity at the time of oocyte pick-up.

- Physicians should be aware of the patient's previous infertility treatments and possible challenges during embryo transfers.
- In case of abdominal ultrasound-guided ET, the patient has to be informed in advance that a full bladder is required.

To Be Prepared on the Day before Transfer

- Prepare a center-well dish with culture medium in the center well and medium in the outer ring (to stabilize the temperature) and without oil for embryo transfer, and incubate overnight at proper gas concentration.

Preparation on the Day

- In case of strictures or malformations within the cervix/uterine cavity premedication with magnesium, scopolamine butylbromide or diclofenac is recommended.
- Patients with transvaginal ultrasound-guided ET should void their bladder before ET.
- The vaginal ultrasound probe must be covered with a special cover (non-sterile) during embryo transfer (ET) and the probe must be cleaned afterwards.
- The embryo(s) must be transferred into the center-well transfer dish before transfer and incubated until transfer.

Embryo Transfer

- ET should be performed in close collaboration with the embryologist.
- All staff members should wear gloves (non-powder).
- Identify patient and embryos provided with patient name.

- Inexperienced physicians should start with transabdominal ultrasound-guided ET.
- Before ET, the procedure itself has to be explained in a comprehensible way to the patient.
- Patient should be in a dorsal position with bent knees and feel comfortable before the procedure is started.
- Talk to the patient and help her to relax and breathe easily throughout the ET.
- Use a soft echogenic catheter.
- Insert a sterile Collin vaginal speculum.
- Expose the cervix and gently clean it with a sterile gauze pad (first 1–2 gauze pads with sterile water and then 1–2 dry gauze pads).
- Remove cervical mucus with a dry gauze pad.
- Insert the outer sheath of the soft embryo catheter.
- Place the ultrasound probe in the vagina or on the abdomen (symphysis).
- Inform the embryologist that the outer sheath of the embryo catheter is placed and that the ET can take place immediately.
- If having trouble during catheter placement, choose another embryo catheter with a rigid outer sheath or try to mold the outer sheath in such a way that it can be inserted in the cervix (e.g., crescent).
- Outer sheath is fixed by the physician until the embryologist places the inner soft catheter.
- Embryologist places the embryo in the soft echogenic inner catheter between two air bubbles using an appropriate culture medium for transfer.
- Embryologist inserts the inner catheter in the outer sheath.
- Transfer depth of the embryo should be in the midportion of the uterus 5–15 mm from the fundal endometrial surface.
- Physician controls transfer depth via transvaginal or transabdominal ultrasound and indicates to the embryologists when the optimal transfer position is reached (ET catheter is placed in the right way).
- Embryologist inserts the embryo steadily with a moderate injection speed followed by pressure on the syringe during slow withdrawal of the catheter.

- Patients can see the echogenic catheter tip on the ultrasound screen as well as air bubbles.
- After transfer the embryologist has to check the outer as well as the inner sheath of the embryo catheter in order to ensure that no embryos were retained.
- Retained embryos should be retransferred using the same technique (ask the patient whether she needs a break before retransfer).
- Patients remains in a reclined position for 10–30 min.
- After the ET patients should be encouraged to avoid intense physical exercise within the following 2 weeks, eat healthily and skip drinking or smoking.
- Patients should receive a letter indicating stimulation protocol, number of obtained and fertilized oocytes, embryo quality and medical treatment during luteal phase.

BIBLIOGRAPHY

Bodri, D., M. Colodrón, D. García, A. Obradors, V. Vernaeve, and O. Coll. 2011. "Transvaginal Versus Transabdominal Ultrasound Guidance for Embryo Transfer in Donor Oocyte Recipients: A Randomized Clinical Trial." *Fertility and Sterility* 95(7): 2263–8, 2268.el.

Rovei, V., P. Dalmasso, G. Gennarelli, T. Lantieri, G. Basso, C. Benedetto, and A. Revelli. "IVF Outcome Is Optimized When Embryos Are Replaced Between 5 and 15 mm From the Fundal Endometrial Surface: A Prospective Analysis on 1184 IVF Cycles." *Reproductive Biology and Endocrinology* 11: 114.

Teixeira, D.M., L.A. Dassunção, C.V. Vieira, M.A. Barbosa, M.A. Coelho Neto, C.O. Nastri, and W.P. Martins. 2015. "Ultrasound Guidance During Embryo Transfer: A Systematic Review and Meta-Analysis of Randomized Controlled Trials." *Ultrasound in Obstetrics & Gynecology* 45(2): 139–48.

Tiras, B., U. Korucuoglu, M. Polat, A. Saltik, H.B. Zeyneloglu, and H. Yarali. 2012. "Effect of Air Bubble Localization After Transfer on Embryo Transfer Outcomes." *European Journal of Obstetrics and Gynecology and Reproductive Biology* 164(1): 52–4.

26

Hygienic Standards in the IVF Laboratory

Vera Baukloh

Principles

Compliance with Legal and/ or Professional Standards

- Hygienic precautions at every step of a treatment by assisted reproduction techniques are part of the risk and safety management and need to be considered in the view of ensuring safety for patients and their gametes and embryos, as well as for staff members.
- There are different legal and/or professional standards with regard to hygiene requirements in every medical procedure in every country, which have to be taken into account.
- For IVF techniques, special emphasis lies on the application of appropriate disinfectants that verifiably do not harm gametes and embryos. This may cause discussions with regulatory bodies but is of vital importance in the field of IVF techniques.

Potential Sources of Risks During the Treatment Cycle

- Carryover of bacterial or viral contamination may occur at any stage during oocyte retrieval, sperm preparation, insemination, handling of oocytes and embryos, cryo-preservation procedures and storage, and embryo transfer.
- Appropriate measures have to be instituted at every step to reliably prevent this without interfering with the workflow.

General Hygienic Precautions

- The lab floor has to be covered with smooth surface material that sustains disinfection.
- During routine work cleaning with water or a mild detergent is advisable.
- For disinfection procedures after spilling or contamination, all human gametes and embryos have to be secured within incubators.

- Perform floor disinfection during work-free intervals to avoid potential hazards to the biological samples.
- Restrict access to the lab to authorized persons in order to avoid introduction of contaminations.
- Use a dedicated changing area adjacent or close to the lab.
- Use appropriate clothing specific for that working area before entering the lab.
- Use special shoes in the lab that are resistant to regular sanitizing procedures.

Protective Precautions for Staff Members

- Get information on the infectious state of the patients on the daily schedule in advance and take specific precautions where reasonable.
- Wear sterile powder-free gloves and face masks—especially while working with body fluids (follicular fluid, semen specimen).
- Disinfect hands before putting gloves on, and after removing gloves, with appropriate disinfectant (not gamete or embryo toxic).
- Avoid mouth-controlled pipetting whenever possible.
- Avoid using sharp material (glass pipettes, cannulas) to prevent injuries.
- Dispose all consumables in an appropriate manner in compliance with legal requirements.
- Do not wear rings, bracelets or necklaces during work in the lab.
- Long hair needs to be tied together or covered with a sterile cap. Bearded male staff members should be encouraged to wear a face mask during all lab procedures.

Consumables and Media Intended for Application in IVF Procedures

- All material and media to be used in handling, culturing or transferring human gametes or embryos have to be sterile and non-toxic.
- The results of all tests performed should be available from the suppliers.
- All IVF media have to contain efficient antibiotics. For prolonged culture a change of medium in-between may be appropriate to ensure that the potency of the antibiotic is not diminishing.

Sterility Problem with an Incubator

Whenever contamination of an incubator is suspected, that respective incubator may not be used until it has once again been made (and proven) aseptic.

Preparation of Working Areas

- Have as few objects as possible on working areas to reduce accumulation of particles.
- Before starting the daily schedule, clean areas and equipment with wipes (not sprays!) soaked in non-toxic disinfectant.
- Between procedures, clean with sterile water. If spilling of body fluids occurs, use disinfectant wipes again, but make sure that all gametes and embryos are accommodated in incubators before starting.
- If a class II flow cabinet is available, do all handling of gametes/embryos within that bench.
- If the lab is equipped with class I cabinets, have the flow working at highest power before starting to work, and switch it off during handling procedures to avoid negative effects of the air stream.
- After finishing all daily work, areas should be decontaminated again.

Basic Precautions During Routine IVF Procedures

Ejaculate Collection

- Have washing facilities for the patients within or close to the room for obtaining sperm.
- Provide a device with hand disinfectant to be used before and after production of the specimen.
- Instruct the patient on appropriate washing procedures for genitalia before starting, and show how to handle the sterile container for the procedure.
- Have all relevant steps in written form also, in case the patient is too nervous to listen.

Insemination of Oocytes

- In case of IVF, add an aliquot of the sperm suspension to the oocytes by means of a sterile pipette or tip.
- In case of ICSI, perform the procedure within medium droplets (with antibiotics) that are covered with warmed sterile mineral oil. Use sterile capillaries only for injecting the single sperm.

Nitrogen for Cryo Preservation/Cryo-Storage

- Work that entails direct contact of samples with liquid nitrogen requires sterilization beforehand by applying UV light, filtration, or comparable effective methods.
- If non-sealed cryo-vessels are used routinely, potentially infected material has to be stored in a quarantine cryo-container.

Protective Measure in Cases of Known Infection in One Partner of an IVF Couple

If there is an infection of bacterial origin in one or both partners, delay IVF treatment until appropriate antibiotics therapy has improved the condition.

Known Infection in the Male Partner

If a treated viral infection is present, perform a sperm preparation before the actual planned treatment cycle by density gradient centrifugation and subsequent washing steps.

- Wear gloves and face mask during the whole procedure.
- Be careful when removing and discarding supernatants to avoid re-introduction of potential virus particles to the prepared sperm suspension.
- All used material and supernatants have to be treated as infectious waste and must be disposed of appropriately.
- Have an aliquot of the sample tested for the actual viral load and cryopreserve the rest in sealed cryo-vessels (store in quarantine!).
- If the aliquot tests negative, the frozen sample is thawed and used to inseminate the female partner's oocytes, preferably by ICSI.

Known Infection in the Female Partner

In case of viral infection in the female, arrange with the clinicians to put that patient on the end of the daily schedule—for oocyte pick-up as well as for transfer.

- Allocate a single incubator to that one patient.
- Perform all handlings with gloves and face mask on.

- Collect all consumables and remnants of used media and dispose of it as infectious waste.
- After the cycle is ended, disinfect the applied incubator thoroughly before using it for other patients.

If many such patients are regularly treated in a facility, a separate lab and dedicated equipment are highly advisable.

Periodical Tests to Verify Hygienic Conditions in the Laboratory

- Microbiological tests have to be performed for the ambient air inside the laboratory and on all relevant equipment in use.
- The frequency may be adjusted to the general findings, i.e., less frequent when the tests are predominantly negative, and more frequent if not.
- Contact plates are preferable for all surfaces like flow-benches and trays inside incubators, while sedimentation plates are adequate for testing the ambient air and the atmosphere inside incubators. If tests are positive, the identification of the germ plus sensitivity testing for antibiotics is mandatory in order to choose the proper disinfectant.

- After every incidence of contamination, the test has to be repeated after decontamination to show the effectiveness of the procedure. Only if the test is negative may the equipment be reintroduced.

BIBLIOGRAPHY

Barnhart, N., M. Shannon, S. Weber, and D. Cohan. 2009. "Assisted Reproduction for Couples Affected by Human Immunodeficiency Virus in California." *Fertility and Sterility* 91: 1540–3.

Magli, M.C., E. Van den Abbeel, K. Lundin, D. Royere, J. Van der Elst, and L. Gianaroli. 2008. "Revised Guidelines for Good Practice in IVF Laboratories." *Human Reproduction* 23: 1253–62.

Mortimer, D. 2004. "A Critical Assessment of the Impact of the European Union Tissue and Cells Directive (2004) on Laboratory Practices in Assisted Conception." *Reproductive BioMedicine Online* 11: 162–76.

Parmegiani, L., A. Accorsi, G.E. Cognigni, S. Bernardi, E. Troilo, and M. Filicori. 2010. "Sterilization of Liquid Nitrogen with Ultraviolet Irradiation for Safe Vitrification of Human Oocytes or Embryos." *Fertility and Sterility* 94: 1525–8.

27

Quality Control of IVF Laboratory Supplies— Mouse Embryo Assay (MEA)

Dean E. Morbeck

Equipment and Supplies

- Waterbath (37°C)
- Test tube rack, timer, stylet, scissors
- Cryopreserved One-cell Murine Embryos, Embryotech Laboratories, Inc.
- Stereo microscope with heated plate
- Heating block for tubes
- CO_2 Incubator at 37°C; CO_2 set to 5%–7% to obtain pH of 7.2–7.3
- 35 mm embryo culture dish
- Stripper pipetter
- Stripper pipette tips (120–150 um diameter)
- Gloves (non-powder)
- A simple salt solution media for embryo culture such as HTF
- HTF-HEPES
- Polyvinyl alcohol (PVA), Sigma P8136–250G
- Light mineral oil
- MEA worksheet

Setup (Day −1)

- Prepare and filter warming (HTF-HEPES; mHTF-PVA) and testing medium (HTF) containing 0.1 mg/mL PVA.
- Prepare 20 μL microdrops of HTF-PVA under mineral oil in a 35 mm culture dish (control). Prepare a minimum of 4 drops: 3 for rinsing and 1 for performing the test.
- Prepare 20 μL microdrops of HTF-PVA exposed to test items (or a different oil) in a separate dish. Prepare a minimum of 4 drops: 3 for rinsing and 1 for performing the test.
- Place prepared dishes in incubator for overnight equilibration.

Setup (Day 0)

- Pre-warm all equipment to the appropriate temperature.
- Pipette 7 mL mHTF-PVA into one 35 mm dish and allow to reach room temperature.
- Prepare workstation near waterbath with timer, test tube rack, stylet, scissors and empty 35 mm dish.

Bioassay Procedure

- A minimum of 10 embryos is required for each test item and the optimal number is 30 per test. Embryos are supplied in groups of 10 or 20 per straw. A reference sheet that comes with each shipment for identifying straws is located in the drawer with QC records.
- Expose the straw to room temperature air for two minutes. Rest the straw horizontally on a test tube rack so that it is surrounded by room temperature air. The straw can be placed anywhere or supported in any way, as long as it rests horizontally and nothing touches the area containing the embryos.
- Place the straw in a 37°C water bath for one minute.
- Remove the straw from the water bath and gently wipe it dry.
- Expel the contents of the straw as a single drop into a sterile 35 mm Petri dish in the following manner: with scissors, remove the lower heat seal. Remove the upper heat seal by cutting to bisect the cotton plug at the PVA section. Using the stylet, push down on the remaining cotton plug expelling the contents of the straw into a sterile Petri dish. To make sure no liquid remains, push the plug to the very end of the straw.
- Using embryo handling pipette (Stripper tip) and working quickly, pick up all embryos in the drop and transfer to room temperature mHTF-PVA. Place embryos at top of media, allowing to sink to rest on

the bottom of the dish. Leave embryos undisturbed at room temperature for 10 minutes.

- Rinse the Stripper tip thoroughly in mHTF-PVA and proceed to transfer embryos in groups of 10 or more to the test dishes while working on a heated stage.

- Expel embryos in first rinse drop, then expel the remainder of mHTF-PVA into the thaw dish.

- Pick up fresh HTF-PVA from the next rinse drop, then move the embryos from the first to the second drop. Repeat the previous two steps until the final drop.

- Using zoom or an inverted microscope, view the embryos to determine the number of viable zygotes. Record total and time on MEA worksheet.

- Assess embryo development at 24, 48, 72, 96, 120 and 144 h post thawing.

- The quality control standard is >75% development to the blastocyst and/or hatching blastocyst stage at 96 hours for 1-cell assay. An enhanced assay is used for mineral oil, where >50% of embryos should remain as expanded blastocysts at 144 h.

- If the standard is not met, retest. After two failed tests, notify the Laboratory Director. Items failing two tests will be discarded and not used for patient purposes.

BIBLIOGRAPHY

Ackerman, S.B., S.P. Taylor, R.J. Swanson, and L.H. Laurell. 1984. "Mouse Embryo Culture for Screening in Human IVF." *Archives of Andrology* 12(Suppl): 129–36.

Gardner, D.K., L. Reed, D. Linck, C. Sheehan, and M. Lane. 2005. "Quality Control in Human in Vitro Fertilization." *Seminars in Reproductive Medicine* 23: 319–24.

Hughes, P.M., D.E. Morbeck, S. Hudson, J. Fredrickson, D.L. Walker, and C.C. Coddington. 2010. "Peroxides in Mineral Oil Used for in Vitro Fertilization: Defining Limits of Standard Quality Control Assays." *Journal of Assisted Reproduction and Genetics* 27: 87–92.

Morbeck, D.E. 2012. "Importance of Supply Integrity for in Vitro Fertilization and Embryo Culture." *Seminars in Reproductive Medicine* 30: 182–90.

Wolff, H.S., J.R. Fredrickson, D.L. Walker, D.E. Morbeck. 2013. "Advances in Quality Control: Mouse Embryo Morphokinetics Are Sensitive Markers of in Vitro Stress." *Human Reproduction* 28: 1776–82.

28

Troubleshooting in the IVF Laboratory

David Mortimer and Sharon T. Mortimer

Principles

- The ability to effectively troubleshoot problems should be an essential skill for anyone who works in an IVF laboratory.
- Application of scientific method is fundamental in troubleshooting, and involves analyzing the various lab processes as well as identifying and measuring both internal and extrinsic factors that control or affect each process.
- Troubleshooting requires a thorough understanding of the basic science of each process: not just the biology, but also the chemistry, physics and engineering upon which the process depends. Without such knowledge the ability to minimize or eliminate problems will be greatly compromised—this is why it is so important when teaching someone a method that one takes the time to explain "why" things are done the way they are, and also often why they are not done in a certain way. Just teaching someone "how" to do something will not produce a truly competent scientist.
- In the context of this chapter, troubleshooting does not include the investigation and analysis of a "one-off" event such as a serious adverse incident.

The Importance of Process

- Effective troubleshooting depends on one's ability to see anything that is done in the IVF laboratory as a process—which is exactly how everything should have been organized from the outset: all IVF laboratory activities must be structured and organized for efficiency and efficacy.
- Process management is simply how one visualizes (e.g., using process mapping), understands, and analyzes how something is done: both how it was intended to be done and how it is actually done.
- Process control provides the essential information on
  - How the process operates normally:
    - Internal control factors.
    - Historical performance, based on one or more key performance indicators (KPIs).
    - Inherent variability (of the KPIs).
    - Extrinsic factors.
    - Uncertainty of measurement (of each KPI).
  - What the process is capable of (based on the KPI(s)):
    - Minimum standards = "competence".
    - Benchmarks = "best practice", based on the proof of the possible.

How to Troubleshoot

- Root cause analysis (RCA) is the standard retrospective risk management tool used as a framework for troubleshooting, and depends on being able to visualize the problem within the context of one or more processes (Mortimer and Mortimer, 2015).
- In any troubleshooting exercise, the following general areas of concern must always be considered:
  - Biological:
    - Patient factors, e.g., atypical age distribution, aberrant case mix or change in referral pattern, unusual pathophysiology.
    - Treatment factors, e.g., stimulation pharmacological responses, inadequate luteal phase support, undiagnosed sperm dysfunction.
  - Organizational:
    - Management choices, e.g., treatment protocol choice, poor criteria for deciding IVF vs. ICSI.
    - Timing, e.g., trigger time, delays in sperm washing, ICSI stripping/injection time, observation or assessments.
  - Technical:
    - Medical procedural aspects, e.g., allowing follicular fluid to cool during oocyte retrieval, trainee with poor ET technique.

- Laboratory procedural aspects, e.g., temperature or pH shifts during gamete or embryo handling and/or assessment.
- Contact materials, e.g., needles and catheters, plasticware, handling devices, culture media.
- Failures or errors, e.g., suboptimal methodology, poor SOPs, unauthorized method change in laboratory SOP.
  - Extrinsic:
    - Macro-environmental factors, e.g., lab design/construction, air quality (especially volatile organic compounds or VOCs).
    - Micro-environmental factors, e.g., workstation and incubator operation.
  - Random chance.
- The overall troubleshooting process is summarized in Table 28.1.

Additional Guidance

During the investigation stage, look at the process in terms of what goes in/what happens to it/what comes out. It is vital that one keeps an open mind—do not make assumptions or jump to conclusions.

When preparing the action plan and writing the report, discuss (possible) "contributory factors", and avoid using the words "cause" or "fault", for legal and psychological reasons. Also, in the report, identify roles generically, do not name individuals.

BIBLIOGRAPHY

Alpha Scientists in Reproductive Medicine. 2015. "The Alpha Consensus Meeting on the professional status of the clinical embryologist: proceedings of an expert meeting." *Reproductive Biomedicine Online* in press.

Mortimer, S.T., and D. Mortimer. *Quality and Risk Management in the IVF Laboratory.* Cambridge: Cambridge University Press, 2015.

TABLE 28.1

Overview of the Troubleshooting Process.

Stage	Action	Specifics
Perception	There is perceived to be a problem	Someone raises a concern that "there seems to be a problem" or "something seems to be wrong"
Inspection	Define the possible problem	Define the review specification: • Identify the particular issue • Identify pertinent KPIs • Establish benchmarks
Verification	Establish that there really is a problem	Review and analyze the KPIs
Investigation	Perform an RCA	Inspect all aspects of the clinic's operations (not just the IVF lab) that could impact on the underlying process(es)
		Audit results, manuals, policies, and the actual performed processes
		Identify possible contributory factors; if it is unclear whether something is contributory, then investigate further (perhaps via the prospective collection of additional data, or even through experimentation)
		Develop a risk matrix of the possible contributory factors
Remediation	Develop an action plan	Plan the likely effective change(s)
		Educate and train all staff as necessary
		Identify suitable KPIs and benchmarks to monitor the change(s)
		Project the improvement(s) that will be achieved = target(s)
		Define a timeline for the change(s) and follow-up
	Effect change	Implement the change(s)
Confirmation	Follow up on the action(s) taken	Based on the projected timeline, monitor the effectiveness of the change(s) using the KPI(s) and appropriate statistical testing
	Review the effectiveness of the action(s) taken	Compare the achieved improvement(s) against the target(s): • Target(s) achieved: Troubleshooting complete, proceed to documentation stage • Target(s) not (all) achieved: Troubleshooting is not complete, return to the inspection stage and repeat
Documentation	Prepare a formal written report on the whole exercise	Essential content: • Document all the actions taken at each stage • Tabulate all data and include statistical analyses • State final conclusion(s)
	Report authorization	Review and acceptance by the Quality Committee
		Report entered into the organization's Quality Manual

29

Microscopy

Markus Montag

Microscope Types Used in IVF

- Stereo microscopes are used for isolation of cumulus oocyte complexes, hyaluronidase treatment, loading and unloading of oocytes and embryos into culture dishes, insemination of oocytes with sperm and embryo transfer.
- Upright light microscopes are used for sperm assessment.
- Inverted light microscopes are used for morphological assessment (sperm, oocytes, zygotes and embryos), IMSI, ICSI, biopsy (polar bodies/blastomeres/trophectoderm cells), assisted hatching and laser manipulation (sperm immobilization, sperm viability testing, biopsy, assisted hatching).

General Microscope Tips and Trouble Shooting

Some microscope types have numerous filters and beam splitters. Make sure that the correct ones are used as wrong positioning does influence image quality, clarity, brightness and overall visibility.

- If you get no image in the eyepiece, check first to see if you can see light coming from the light source.
  - If there is no light: check the bulb and, if necessary, replace the bulb (*Caution:* bulb may be hot).
  - If there is light: check filters and beam splitters, as there may be a wrong setting.
- If you get no image on a screen: check the light source, check camera power, check the beam splitter position(s), check cable connection from camera to screen.
- Always keep a replacement bulb close to a microscope (make sure to use the correct type as it may differ for different microscopes). along with the instructions on how to change a bulb.

- Any parts that can become dusty need to be cleaned at regular intervals, preferably by using an air blower.
- Always try to protect the front lens of the objectives from scratches, dust etc.

Microscope Adjustment

- Adjustment requires knowledge about the light path in the microscope. All inverted and standard microscopes have a light source, various filters, a light source aperture, a condenser with adjustable settings and a condenser aperture, the specimen holder/plane, several objectives, mirrors and beam splitter(s), 1–2 eyepieces/oculars, and a camera port.
- Major adjustments that must be done regularly:
  - Adjust the eyepieces/oculars according to the strength of your eyes (dioptry).
  - Adjust the correct illumination of the specimen as follows: close the light source aperture, visualize the aperture by looking through the eyepieces, focus the aperture by changing the height position of the condenser, then center the aperture by using the center-aid at the condenser and open the aperture so that it just disappears out of the field of view (this procedure is called "Köhler adjustment").
- For some objectives, the thickness of the cover slip/bottom of the dish between the specimen and the objective can be adjusted at a ring on the objective.

Special Microscope Technologies and Adjustments

Phase Contrast

- Use a 20× or 40× phase objective.
- Set the condenser to the proper phase ring, remove one eyepiece to visualize the phase rings from the objective and the condenser in the tubes.

- Adjust the phase rings so that both match.
- Repeat for other objectives.
- Some microscopes come with a visualization aid that fits into the eyepiece holder.

Hoffman Contrast (HC)/Differential Interference Contrast (DIC)

- This mode requires a prism in the objective and a prism in the condenser.
  - For DIC, both can be adjusted. For HC, usually only the condenser prism can be adjusted.
  - Different condenser prisms are used for different purposes (use correct setting).
- Always chose a setting that gives an illumination on the screen/image from the upper left as this is our natural perception of illumination.
- In general, use a setting that gives a high contrast at a close to uniform illumination.
- Original DIC requires glass bottom dishes/slides.

Laser-Adapted Microscope

- Lasers (e.g., for zona opening/sperm immobilization) are adapted either through assembly of the laser diode unit at the fluorescence port or through an objective.
- Delivery of the laser beam to the specimen depends on:
  - The type of objective (must be suitable for the laser wavelength).
  - Mirrors and filters in the beam path (some may block the laser).
  - The distance the laser travels through water (culture medium).
  - The culture media composition.

High Magnification Microscopy as for MSOME/IMSI

- The original setup uses a 100× DIC objective and requires immersion oil between the objective and a flat glass bottom dish.
  - Settings are adjusted as described for DIC.
- A computer-adapted setup requires a 60× objective without oil but setting of dish bottom thickness.

Polarization Microscopy

- This mode requires a polarizer behind the light source and an analyzer behind the condenser.
- In standard polarization microscopy (e.g., that used for sperm birefringence), both can be adjusted and usually are crossed to eliminate normal light and allow polarized light to pass.
- For spindle and zona imaging in oocytes, systems are used where a circumpolar polarizer is used together with a computer-controlled analyzer.
  - This requires no adjustment but a green filter for illumination.
- Polarized microscopy only works with glass bottom dishes or slides.

Time-Lapse Microscopy

- There are two types of time-lapse microscopes.
  - One is a special microscope that is built into an incubation system to form an integrated time-lapse system for incubation under constant imaging of embryos. The time intervals for image assembly, the numbers of focal planes and the distance between the focal planes have to be adjusted prior to initiation of an imaging cycle by computer software.
  - The other is a stand-alone microscope that can be placed into an incubator. Settings are adjusted via computer software.

BIBLIOGRAPHY

Montag M., R. Klose, M. Köster, B. Rösing, K. van der Ven, K. Rink, and H. van der Ven. 2009. "Application of Non-Contact Laser Technology in Assisted Reproduction." *Medical Laser Application* 24: 57–64.

Montag, M., M. Köster, K. van der Ven, and H. van der Ven. 2011. "Gamete Competence Assessment by Polarization Microscopy." *Human Reproduction Update* 17: 654–66.

Montag, M., K.S. Pedersen, and N.B. Ramsing. "Time Lapse Imaging of Embryo Development: Using Morphokinetic Analysis to Select Viable Embryos." In *Culture Media, Solutions, and Systems in Human ART*, edited by P. Quinn, 518–36. Cambridge: Cambridge University Press, 2014.

30

Fertility Preservation

Markus Montag and Jana Liebenthron

Methods of Fertility Preservation Prior Gonadotoxic Therapy

- Cryopreservation of spermatozoa/testicular tissue after preparation (Chapters 8 and 14).
- Cryopreservation of oocytes and/or embryos after hormone stimulation (Chapter 15).
- **Note:** Embryo cryopreservation has challenges in case of divorce.
- Cryopreservation of ovarian tissue.
- **Note:** This chapter only describes sperm/TESE and ovarian tissue freezing. For oocyte/embryo freezing, refer to Chapter 15.

Required Equipment

- Setup for individual procedures as described in Chapters 3, 6, 8, 10, 11, 14, 15
- Sperm freeze medium (SFM)
- Liquid nitrogen
- Nitrogen dewar container
- Storage tank (vapor phase/liquid phase)
- Programmable freezer
- Ovarian tissue preparation medium
- Sterile scalpels and forceps
- Cooling plate
- Cryo-tubes
- Security equipment for handling liquid nitrogen
- Documentation chart

To Be Prepared on the Day before (Sperm Freezing/Ovarian Tissue Freezing)

- For sperm/TESE, preparation as described in Chapters 8 and 14
- For ovarian tissue: suitable medium for transportation, preparation and cryopreservation, all to be stored at 4°C

Preparation on the Day (Sperm Freezing/Ovarian Tissue Freezing)

- Prepare for sperm/TESE preparation as described in Chapters 8 and 14.
- For ovarian tissue:
  - Hand over the tube with the transportation medium to the surgery team with proper instruction on tissue handling.
  - Pre-fill cryotubes with cold (4°C) ovarian tissue cryopreservation medium.

Sperm Pre-freezing Procedure (Native Ejaculate/Prepared Sperm)

- For freezing of native ejaculate, let the ejaculate liquefy.
- For freezing of prepared sperm, dissolve sperm preparation in a suitable volume of sperm preparation medium.
- Determine the volume for freezing and pipette into a 13–15 mL tube.
- Fill a syringe with the appropriate volume of sperm freeze medium.
- Drop SFM slowly, and while swirling the tube, into the ejaculate.
- **Note:** Some SFM are added in the ratio 1 part of SFM to 1 volume part of ejaculate, others 0.7 part of SFM to 1 volume part of ejaculate.
- Distribute SFM/ejaculate mix to labeled cryo-tubes.

Testicular Tissue Pre-freezing Procedure

- Wear gloves.
- Pre-fill cryo-tubes with sperm freezing medium/room temperature (RT).
- Identify patient/material provided with patient name/label tubes.

- Dissect TESE material into small pieces and transfer pieces into pre-filled cryo-tubes.
- Equilibrate cryo-tubes for 30 min at RT.
- [*Optional:* Perform sperm preparation from TESE tissue preparation as described in Chapter 14 and proceed to sperm freezing for the TESE sperm suspension.]

Freezing Procedure for Ejaculate/ Prepared Sperm/Testicular Tissue

- Freeze cryo-tubes with freezing mix (SFM plus ejaculate, sperm, tissue) with a suitable program in a programmable slow freezer.
- [*Optional:* Freeze cryo-tubes in nitrogen vapor by placing the tubes approximately 8–10 cm above liquid nitrogen in a dewar container; cover with a loose fitting plate.]

Sperm (Frozen Prepared Sperm/ Ejaculate) Thawing

- Remove cryo-tubes from storage tank.
- Place tubes in warm water (37°C) until ice is just melted completely.
- Remove the entire volume and place in a centrifuge tube (for frozen native ejaculate, continue directly with sperm preparation by gradient centrifugation—see Chapter 8).
- Add to 1–2 mL of volume 3 mL of sperm preparation medium and mix gently.
- Centrifuge at 300–350 g for 15 min and discard supernatant.
- For frozen prepared sperm: Dissolve pellet in a suitable medium and at a suitable volume for insemination, IVF or ICSI.

Testicular Tissue Thawing

- Remove cryo-tubes from storage tank.
- Place tubes in warm water (37°C) until ice is just melted completely.
- Remove tissue pieces and place in a centrifuge tube with warm sperm preparation medium (37°C) to facilitate cryo-medium exchange.
- Perform sperm preparation from tissue as described in Chapter 14.

Ovarian Tissue Freezing

- Retrieve tissue from surgical team.

- Work for preparation in an aseptic environment (preferably Lamina class A in a clean room).
- Wear gloves.
- Identify patient/material provided with patient name/label tubes.
- Retrieve tissue from transportation tube and place into a dish containing preparation medium that is placed on a cooling plate (approximately 4°C).
- Use scalpels and forceps to remove gently stroma tissue from the cortex.
- Prepare a thin cortex layer (1–2 mm thick), leaving a tender layer of the medulla on the cortex surface.
- Cut cortex into pieces (6–8 × 5 mm).
- Pre-equilibrate pieces in a container with cryo-preservation medium for 20 min at 4°C (preferably under constant agitation).
- Transfer pieces into pre-cooled cryotubes pre-filled with cryopreservation medium.
- Place cryotubes in a suitable programmable freezer.
- Equilibrate for another 10 min at 4°C prior to start of the slow freezing program.
- Perform seeding at −6°C to −8°C.
- Transfer cryotubes to storage tank after end of program (end temperature < −180°C).

Ovarian Tissue Thawing Prior Re-transplantation

- Perform all steps in an aseptic environment (see above).
- Prepare sterile filtrated thawing solutions (20 mL each 0.75 M, 0.375 M, 0.125 M sucrose in D-PBS, 10% HSA).
- Remove cryotubes with appropriate number of tissue pieces for immediate transplantation from storage tank.
- Place tubes in warm water (37°C) until ice is just (but not completely) melted.
- Remove tissue pieces and place in a container with 0.5 M thawing solution for 15–20 min under constant agitation at RT.
- Transfer pieces to 0.25 M followed by 0.125 M thawing solution followed by D-PBS with 10% HSA for 15–20 min each.
- Transfer to a tube with D-PBS and 10% HSA and immediately transport to the surgery room for immediate transplantation.

BIBLIOGRAPHY

Bastings, L., J. Liebenthron, J.R. Westphal, C.C.M. Beerendonk, H. van der Ven, B. Meinecke, M., D.D.M. Braat, and R. Peek. 2014. "Efficacy of Ovarian Tissue Freezing in a Major European Center." *Journal of Assisted Reproduction & Genetics* 31: 1003–12.

Liebenthron, J., and M. Montag. "Development of a Nationwide Network for Ovarian Tissue Cryopreservation." In *Gamete and Embryo Cryopreservation: Methods and Protocols*, edited by A. Agarwal, Z.P. Nagy, and A. Varghese. New York: Springer, 2017; in press.

Liebenthron, J., J. Reinsberg, K. van der Ven, H. van der Ven, M. Köster, M. Kühr, and M. Montag. 2015. "Fertility Preservation Using Ovarian Tissue: 10 Years Experience From a Centralized Cryobanking Facility in Germany." In preparation for submission.

von Wolff, M., M. Montag, R. Dittrich, D. Denschlag, F. Nawroth, and B. Lawrenz. 2011. "Fertility Preservation in Women—A Practical Guide of Preservation Techniques and Therapeutic Strategies in Breast Cancer, Hodgkin's Lymphoma and Borderline Ovarian Neoplasms." *Archives of Gynecology and Obstetrics* 284: 427–35.

Section II

Clinical Procedures

31

Ultrasound Evaluation in Treatment Management

Ippokratis Sarris and Geeta Nargund

Equipment

- Gynecological examination couch with stirrups
- Ultrasound machine with both a transvaginal transducer (between 5–9 MHz) and an abdominal transducer (3.5–5 MHz)
- Ultrasound gel to facilitate acoustic coupling [*Optional:* with warmer]
- Transducer covers (latex and non-latex)
- Gowns or sheets for women to change into or cover themselves (disposable or washable)
- Examination gloves (latex and/or non-latex)
- Faucet and basin for handwashing
- Female chaperone

Before Starting the Ultrasound Evaluation

- Ask the woman if she has emptied her bladder and if she is allergic to latex, then choose the appropriate gloves and transducer cover.
- Explain to the woman what you are going to do and why.
- Request for a female chaperone to be present during the procedure.
- Ask the woman to remove her clothes from the waist down, cover herself with a gown or sheet and sit at the end of the examination couch in private.
- Wash your hands and wear gloves.
- Place a small amount of gel inside the probe cover (usually 2–3 mL should suffice) and insert the ultrasound probe in the cover, which should be rolled down all the way to the handle. Ensure that no air is trapped between the top of the probe and the inside of the cover, as this will reduce the acoustic coupling and lead to image artifacts.
- Place a similar amount of gel on the outside of the cover, on the top of the transducer.

Performing the Ultrasound Evaluation

- Ask the woman to lie down on the examination couch with her legs in the stirrups and her bottom at the edge of the bed (**Note:** If the woman is too high up the bed, probe movements will be restricted as the end of the bed will impede with the full range of movements required).
- Keep her as minimally exposed as possible.
- Give warning when the examination is about to start and encourage her to inform you if she finds it uncomfortable.
- Gently insert the ultrasound transducer in the vagina and all the way up to the cervix.
- At this stage, it is assumed that the woman has already had a thorough initial scan to assess the pelvic organs, therefore at this stage the ultrasound evaluation is targeted at findings that are relevant to guiding the management of ongoing fertility treatment.
- There are three main areas that need to be evaluated systematically:
  - Uterus.
  - Ovaries.
  - Remainder of pelvis.

Uterine Evaluation

- A mid-Sagittal view of the uterus should be acquired in order to visualize the endometrium.
- Measure the endometrial thickness by placing calipers perpendicular to the midline echo, at the thickest point. The calipers should be placed at the junctions of the endometrium and the myometrium.
- Assess the appearance of the endometrium—menstrual, triple layer, intermediate or hyper-echogenic.
- Look for the presence of any focal echogenic areas (suggestive of a polyp or fibroid).
- Look for the presence of fluid (in the absence of menses, this is suggestive of intrauterine adhesions, a communicating hydrosalpinx or infection).

- Pan throughout the uterus, both in longitudinal and transverse planes, to visualize the entire endometrium and myometrium.
- Comment on the presence of any myometrial abnormalities such as fibroids, adenomyosis, or abnormal shape of the cavity.
- *Optional:* Color Doppler studies of the uterine arteries and subendometrial vessels.

Ovarian Evaluation

- Locate either of the ovaries first in the transverse plane.
- Pan throughout the ovary and count the overall number of follicles (all follicles measuring 2 mm and above).
- Start from one end of the ovary and systematically measure each follicle separately.
- Follicles are usually measured in two orthogonal dimensions (inner wall to inner wall).
  - However, as many may be ellipsoid, if only two dimensions are measured then the resultant average diameter might be misleading.
  - Therefore, for leading follicles and follicles measuring more than 10 mm, taking the mean of all three dimensions is more accurate.
  - This requires imaging the ovary both in the transverse and the longitudinal plane.
- Look for the presence of any other features/abnormalities such as a corpus luteum or cysts.
- If an abnormal structure is found, then characterize it by: measuring its size in three dimensions; commenting on the echogenicity; assessing if it is cystic, solid or mixed; looking for internal septae and papillary projections; evaluating the vascularity using Doppler flow; mobility and relation to other pelvic structures.
- Comment on the position and mobility of the ovary in relation to the uterus and other pelvic structures for the purpose of access for a transvaginal oocyte retrieval.
  - Assess if the access is anticipated to be transvaginally (and if so easily or with concomitant abdominal pressure and/or probe manipulation). Might a trans-myometrial approach be necessary? Is access possible only transabdominally?
- Repeat the procedure for the contralateral ovary (unless absent).
- *Optional:* Color Doppler studies of the ovarian stromal and peri-follicular vessels, automated follicular measurement algorithms and three-dimensional sonography. These have all been studied widely, however, their use in routine practice is still being evaluated.
- **Note:** Transabdominal ultrasound evaluation of the ovaries with a full bladder might be required if these are not visible vaginally—this can be due to the presence of fibroids; adhesions that have fixed the ovaries above the uterus; transfixing of ovaries at the pelvic brim due to previous oncological treatment. This will also allow assessing if a transabdominal approach to oocyte retrieval is possible.

Remainder of Pelvic Evaluation

- Look at the Pouch of Douglas for free fluid (as this can indicate recent ovulation) or for encapsulated fluid (indicative of pelvic adhesions).
- Look for any adnexal masses and characterize them (in a similar fashion to ovarian masses).
- **Note:** Occasionally, women may be unable to tolerate a transvaginal ultrasound examination due to vaginismus, in which case a transabdominal scan is required.

Finishing the Ultrasound Evaluation

- Withdraw the ultrasound transducer and remove its cover, which should be disposed in a clinical waste bag along with the gloves.
- Allow the woman to dress in private.
- Disinfect the ultrasound transducer and clean the bed as per the unit protocol.
- Wash your hands.
- Explain the findings to the woman.
- Discuss plan and next steps in management.
- Record and document clearly the findings and plan.

BIBLIOGRAPHY

Dubey, A.K., H.A. Wang, P. Duffy and A.S. Penzias. 1995. "The Correlation Between Follicular Measurements, Oocyte Morphology, and Fertilization Rates in an in Vitro Fertilization Program." *Fertility and Sterility* 64: 787–90.

Practice Committee of American Society for Reproductive Medicine. 2012. Diagnostic evaluation of the infertile female: a committee opinion. *Fertility and Sterility* 98: 302.

Scheffer, G.J., F.J.M. Broekmans, L.F. Bancsi, J.D.F. Habbema, C.W.N. Looman and E.R. Te Velde. 2002. "Quantitative Transvaginal Two- and Three-Dimensional Sonography of the Ovaries: Reproducibility of Antral Follicle Counts." *Ultrasound in Obstetrics & Gynecology* 20: 270–5.

Raine-Fenning, N., S. Deb, K. Jayaprakasan, J. Clewes, J. Hopkisson et al. 2010. "Timing of Oocyte Maturation and Egg Collection: During Controlled Ovarian Stimulation: a Randomized Controlled Trial Evaluating Manual and Automated Measurements of Follicle Diameter." *Fertility and Sterility* 94: 184–8.

32

Three-Dimensional Ultrasound and the Diagnosis of Uterine Anomalies

Magued Adel Mikhail, Megan Lively, Candice P. Holliday, and Botros Rizk

Introduction

Three-dimensional (3D) ultrasound (US) has the unique capability of assessing both the uterine cavity and fundus, because it has the distinct advantage of demonstrating the coronal plane, which lies perpendicular to the transducer and cannot be obtained by the two-dimensional (2D) scan. Congenital uterine anomalies are common and their effect on fertility and reproductive outcome is significant, hence the importance of accurate diagnosis. The incidence is difficult to establish in asymptomatic women, but it is estimated to be 0.1%–3% of all women. It is prevalent in 2%–8% of the infertile group, in 5%–30% of women who suffered from miscarriages, and in 3%–38% of patients with recurrent miscarriages.

Equipment

- The US room should be private, with an examination table and a cover to keep patient dignity.
- High-frequency US machine with 3D capability and capacity to store and analyze the pictures with 3D vaginal probe.
- Lubricating gel and medical gloves should be available.

Technique

- The US scan should be performed by a fertility specialist, radiologist, or sonographer with experience in 3D technology and the interpretation of results.
- After verbal consent, a systematic 2D examination is started with anatomical orientation of the uterine fundus and cervix.
- The picture is optimized using the gain and depth tool.
- Once a satisfactory longitudinal 2D picture is obtained, the 3D button is activated and the probe

is maintained still. It takes 10 seconds to obtain the volume.
- Throughout the scan the patient should be engaged.
- 3D US is based on one-dimensional transducer arrays whose position is known accurately by position-sensor. Volume acquisition starts by using 2D images with superimposed VOL-box, which frames the region of interest (ROI). The volume scan sweeps from one margin to the other.
- For sectional (multiplanar) navigation, the three images represent the three orthogonal planes (A, B and C).
- The ROI is chosen and included in the VOL box.
- The orientation point in images A and B are adjusted to obtain clear image in C.
- The picture is improved using the VCI (thick slice) tool.
- Parallel shift could be used to get different planes, and omniview is useful when the ROI is curved and the X, Y, and Z buttons are used to rotate the pictures in the three orthogonal planes.
- The Z technique allows easy manipulation of the image to identify the best orientation to see the mid-fundal region of the uterus, both externally and internally.
- The surface rendering option allows visualization of the organ with varying degrees of contrast and light.
- The four images represent A, B, and C as the multiplanar option and the 3D rendered view image.
- The ROI is included in the VOL box, ideally with the green line on top and adjusted.

Classification of Uterine Anomalies

- The American Fertility Society (AFS) classification was first used in 1988 and remains the cornerstone for the classification of uterine anomalies.

- The European Society of Human Reproduction and Embryology (ESHRE) and European Society of Gynecological Endoscopy (ESGE) published another classification in 2013.

Unicornuate Uterus

- A unicornuate uterus occurs when one Müllerian duct develops normally and the other does not, resulting in unilateral hypoplasia or agenesis.
- It can be sub-classified into communicating, no cavity, and no horn.
- In 83% of cases, the rudimentary horn is non-communicating.
- The diagnosis is possible with the 2D scan.
- 3D scan helps the accurate diagnosis with 360-degree assessment for presence of only one cornu.
- Congenital renal malformations are commonly associated.
- Pre-pregnancy counselling, single embryo transfer, and pregnancy complications, including miscarriage and preterm labor, should be discussed.

Didelphic Uterus

- Uterine didelphys is very rare and it occurs when the two Müllerian ducts fail to fuse, thus producing duplication of the reproductive system.
- Generally, the duplication is limited to the uterus and cervix, with uterine didelphys and bicollis (two cervices) or unicollis (one cervix).
- Didelphic uterus and bicollis often have good reproductive outcomes.

Bicornuate Uterus

- Bicornuate uterus results from only partial fusion of the Müllerian ducts.
- This results in a variable degree of separation of the uterine horns that can be complete or partial.
- Typically, there is only one cervix and two endometrial cavities.

- The patient should be counselled about cervical incompetence and preterm labor.

Septate Uterus

- The septate uterus is strongly associated with pregnancy loss as a result of the poor vascularization of the septum and the presence of fibrous tissue.
- 3D US is accurate in diagnosing septate uterus and has very good agreement with MRI. It can differentiate septate uterus from bicornuate uterus without the need for laparoscopy.
- Hysteroscopic resection of the septum is the standard management.

Arcuate Uterus

- The fundus projects in the cavity to a depth less than 10 mm and normal aerosol surface.
- There is an associated higher incidence of late second and third trimester complications.

BIBLIOGRAPHY

Abuzeid, M. and O. Abuzeid. "Three Dimensional Ultrasonography of Subtle Uterine Anomalies: Correlation with Hysterosalpingogram, Two Dimensional Ultrasonography and Hysteroscopic." In *Ultrasonography in Gynecology*, edited by B. Rizk and E. Puscheck, 66–79. Cambridge: Cambridge University Press, 2015.

Assad, N. and S. Huston. "Three Dimensional Ultrasonography in Gynecology". In *Ultrasonography in Gynecology*, edited by B. Rizk and E. Puscheck, 1–11. Cambridge: Cambridge University Press, 2015.

Awonuga, A.O., S. Johnson, M. Singh, and E. Puscheck. "Mullerian Anomaly and Ultrasonographic Diagnosis." In *Ultrasonography in Gynecology*, edited by B. Rizk and E. Puschec, 43–57. Cambridge: Cambridge University Press, 2015.

Kupesic, S. 2005. "Three Dimensional Ultrasound in Reproductive Medicine." *Ultrasound in Obstetrics and Gynaecology* 5: 304–15.

33

Infertility Ultrasound Evaluation: One-Stop Procedure

Spiros A. Liatsikos and Geeta Nargund

Required Equipment

- High-resolution ultrasound device with a transvaginal transducer, equipped with sensitive color and spectral Doppler modalities, and ideally a three-dimensional (3D) facility
- Latex and non-latex covers for vaginal transducer
- Ultrasound gel
- Additionally, for hydrosonography and/or hysterosalpingo-contrast-sonography (HyCoSy): speculum, balloon catheter or simple intrauterine insemination catheter, and negative (saline) and positive (SonoVue, Bracco International BV, Amsterdam, The Netherlands) contrast medium

Timing of Fertility Ultrasound Scan

Any time, preferably between days 8 and 10 of a 28-day menstrual cycle.

Two Days before the Ultrasound Scan

Start prophylactic antibiotic coverage if hydrosonography and/or HyCoSy are planned. Unless allergies exist, a combination of metronidazole and doxycycline is recommended.

Preparation on the Day

- Set up ultrasound device for gynecological transvaginal scan.
- Input patient's identification details in ultrasound device.
- Place new cover and ultrasound gel on the top of vaginal transducer.
- Prepare and warm contrast medium to room temperature (for HyCoSy).[1]
- Welcome patient and introduce practitioner.

- Ask patient for a brief medical and gynecological history, including if there is allergy to latex, sulphur and sulphur containing products (especially if SonoVue is used for HyCoSy).
- Explain to patient the procedure of the fertility ultrasound scan, the need for it to be transvaginal, and the expected findings.
- Ask for a female staff chaperone.
- Advise patient on how to prepare herself for the scan and sit in a position suitable for transvaginal access.

Performing the Fertility Ultrasound Evaluation

Uterus

- Identify the uterus (present/absent).
- Assess position (antiverted, retroverted, axial).
- Assess mobility.
- Measure dimensions (linear, transverse, anterioposterior).
- Assess morphology. Identify and differentiate congenital malformations (arcuate, subseptate, bicornuate or didelphys uterus), mainly with 3D ultrasound scan.
- Identify and measure fibroids. Assess their position (anterior, posterior, fundal, lateral, cervical), type (pedunculated, subserosal, intramural, submucous), and proximity to endometrium.
- Identify adenomyosis.
- Identify scars from previous operations. Note details of cesarean scar dehiscence if present.
- Assess uterine blood flow. Use Doppler to calculate uterine artery peak systolic velocity (PSV) and pulsatility index (PI).

Endometrium

- Assess outline, morphology (menstrual, early follicular, triple layer, secretory, atrophic, hyperplastic, hyperechogenic) and its accordance with time of cycle.

- Measure thickness.
- Identify and measure polyps and submucosal fibroids.
- Identify mucus in cervical canal.
- Apply color Doppler to visualize vessels (spiral arteries) extending into the endometrium.[2]
- Perform hydrosonography, if needed (see below).

Ovaries

- Identify both ovaries (present/absent).
- Assess position, mobility, and accessibility for potential transvaginal or transabdominal oocyte retrieval.
- Assess morphology (normal, polycystic, multifollicular).
- Measure dimensions and calculate volume.
- Identify, measure, and differentiate cysts (simple, complex, endometrioma, dermoid). Assess cystic and pericystic vascularity using Doppler. Evaluate the risk of ovarian malignancy.
- Identify dominant follicle (follicular phase) or corpus luteum (luteal phase). Measure dimensions and calculate mean diameter and volume of those structures. Assess perifollicular blood flow using Doppler and calculate PSV.[3,4]
- Assess early antral follicle count (AFC 2–5 mm). Measure dimensions and identify late antral follicles (mean diameter >5 mm) for both ovaries.[5]
- Assess stromal blood flow using Doppler and calculate PSV.[6,7]
- Identify and measure para-ovarian cysts.

Fallopian Tubes

- Identify presence of hydrosalpinx and measure its dimensions.
- Assess tubal patency with HyCoSy, if needed (see below).

Pouch of Douglas

- Identify fluid (free, encysted) and estimate its volume.
- Identify masses and their origin.

Hydrosonography and/or HyCoSy

- Insert speculum. Identify cervix and external cervical os.
- Insert a balloon catheter or a simple intrauterine insemination catheter through cervical canal.
- Inject 1 mL saline into the balloon to stabilize the catheter.

- Inject negative contrast (saline) through the catheter until dilatation of the uterine cavity is confirmed with ultrasound scan.
- Assess the mucosa and identify polyps, submucosal fibroids, or endometrial adhesions.
- Inject more saline and apply color Doppler to demonstrate flow through the fallopian tubes.
- Inject 2–5 mL positive contrast (SonoVue) very slowly into each fallopian tube.
- Demonstrate the medium in the fallopian tubes and spill into the peritoneal cavity.
- Identify right/left/bilateral proximal or distal occlusion.[8]
- Aspirate saline from balloon, remove catheter and speculum.

After the Ultrasound Scan

- Provide patient with clean wipes.
- Remove cover and clean thoroughly the vaginal transducer.
- Print ultrasound images and/or save them.
- Prepare a detailed report of all the findings and provide patient with a copy.
- Explain to patient in detail the normal and abnormal findings of her ultrasound scan.
- Suggest further investigations, if needed (hysteroscopy, laparoscopy, etc.).
- Discuss options for treatment and explain the expected chance of success with each type of treatment.
- Advise patient to stay on prophylactic antibiotic coverage for 3 more days if she had hydrosonography and/or HyCoSy.

REFERENCES

1. B. Nirmal, A.N. Griffiths, G. Jose, and J. Evans, "Warming Echovist Contrast Medium for Hystero-Contrast Sonography and the Effect on the Incidence of Pelvic Pain. A Randomized Controlled Study," *Human Reproduction* 21(4) (2006): 1052–4.
2. R. Mona, M. Carine, S. Valerie, et al., "Study of Uterine Spiral Arteries During Implantation Window in Women with Normal Fertility or Implantation Failure," *American Journal of Reproductive Immunology* 60(1) (2008): 87–8.
3. G. Nargund, "Time for an Ultrasound Revolution in Reproductive Medicine," *Ultrasound in Obstetrics & Gynecology* 20 (2002): 107–11.
4. P. Bhal, N. Pugh, D.K. Chui, et al., "The Use of Transvaginal Power Doppler Ultrasonography to Evaluate the Relationship Between Perifollicular Vascularity and Outcome of in-Vitro Fertilisation Treatment Cycles," *Human Reproduction* 14(4) (1999): 919–45.

5. D.J. Hendricks, E.W. Mol, L.F. Banksi, et al., "Antral Follicle Count in the Prediction of Poor Ovarian Response and Pregnancy After Invitro Fertilisation; a Meta Analysis and Comparison with Basal Follicle Stimulating Hormone Level," *Fertility and Sterility* 83(2) (2005): 291–301.

6. L. Engmann, P. Sladkevicius, R. Agrawal, et al., "Value of Ovarian Stromal Blood Flow Velocity Measurement After Pituitary Suppression in the Prediction of Ovarian Responsiveness and Outcome of in Vitro Fertilization Treatment." *Fertility and Sterility* 71(1) (1999): 22–9.

7. J.S. Younis, S. Haddad, M. Matilsky, et al., "Undetectable Basal Ovarian Stromal Blood Flow in Infertile Women Is Related to Low Ovarian Reserve," *Gynecological Endocrinology* 23(5) (2007): 284–9.

8. S. Killick, "Hysterosalpingo-contrast Sonography as a Screening Test for Tubal Patency in Infertile Women," *Journal of the Royal Society of Medicine* 92 (1999): 628–31.

34

Office Hysteroscopy

Linda D. Bradley

Required Equipment

- Hysteroscope options
  - Flexible hysteroscope
  - Rigid hysteroscope
- *Optional:*
  - Camera
  - Video recorder
  - Photography
- Video tower
- Light source
- Variable speculum sizes due to patient parity or weight
- 60 mL syringes filled with sterile saline
- Sterile extension tubing
- Examination table with stirrups or knee braces and ideally able to change position to Trendelenburg position
- *Optional:*
  - Heating pad
  - Pillow
- Emergency equipment
  - Emergency cart
  - Oxygen
  - Spirits of ammonia
  - Contact information for prompt transport if significant vasovagal response

To Be Prepared on the Day Before

- Knowledge of how many anticipated patients, so that the appropriate number of sterile hysteroscopes will be available.
- Ideally, patients would have received written material to instruct them to eat before the procedure and take an NSAID 2–4 hours before the procedure.

Preparation on the Day

- Sterile basin to draw up saline
- Draw up and label 60 mL saline syringes
- Sterile IV extension tubing
- Antiseptic solution for cleansing vagina and cervix (baby shampoo, Betadine, etc.)
- Sterile speculum
- Time out: identify patient name, birthdate, and medical record number
- Obtain vital signs, including blood pressure and pulse
- Obtain urine pregnancy testing and confirm that it is negative
- Informed consent for hysteroscopy and possible endometrial biopsy
- Confirm proper timing (early proliferative phase) of the endometrium
- Explain the procedure to the patient with both written and verbal instructions and answer patient questions, if needed

Procedure

- Put on non-sterile examination gloves and insert speculum. Examine the cervix to exclude mucopurulent discharge or cervicitis. Perform Pap test and HPV testing if clinically indicated.
- Remove the speculum and then perform bimanual exam to determine size, position, and exclude uterine tenderness. If signs of infection, discontinue planned procedure.
- Cleanse cervix with antiseptic solution.
- Change gloves and put on sterile gloves.
- Determine if cervical dilation is needed, depending on the diameter of the hysteroscope used.
- If cervical dilation is needed, use tapered "os finder dilator" or narrow Hegar dilator. Use narrow tooth tenaculum only as needed to stabilize the cervix.

- Remove sterile hysteroscope from case and attach sterile IV tubing and sterile saline syringe and flush the tubing and hysteroscope to remove air from IV tubing.
- Attach camera if using the hysteroscope.
- Insert hysteroscope under direct visualization and slowly push the sterile saline at individualized rate for optimal visualization and patient comfort.
- Carefully inspect the endocervix, endometrial cavity, and tubal ostia.
- Determine if there are congenital uterine anomalies, endometrial polyps, intracavitary leiomyoma, leiomyoma that impinge on uterine cavity, endometrial hyperplasia, or uterine malignancy.
- Based on clinical findings, determine if endometrial biopsy is needed.
- Take photographs of hysteroscopic findings if clinically available.
- Document hysteroscopic findings in the medical record.
- Explain findings to the patient and the clinical plan of care.
- Provide the patient with discharge instructions and details of who to contact if post-procedural pain, fever, or purulent discharge.
- Make follow-up appointment as clinically indicated.

BIBLIOGRAPHY

Bradley, L.D. "Indications and Contraindications for Office Hysteroscopy." In *Hysteroscopy: Office Evaluation and Management of the Uterine Cavity*, edited by L.D. Bradley and T. Falcone. Philadelphia, PA: Mosby, 2009.

Keats, J.P. 2013. "Procedures in the Office Setting Patient Safety in the Obstetric and Gynecology Office Setting." *Obstetrics & Gynecology Clinics of North America* 40: 611–23.

Keyhan, S., and M.G. Munro. 2014. "Office Diagnostic and Operative Hysteroscopy Using Local Anesthesia Only; an Analysis of Patient Reported Pain and Other Procedural Outcomes." *Journal of Minimally Invasive Gynecology* 21(5): 791–8.

35

Hysteroscopic Management of Uterine Septum

Omar Abuzeid and Mostafa Abuzeid

Introduction

Uterine septum accounts for 34%–48% of structural uterine anomalies; the issue of uterine septum and infertility remains controversial. This Müllerian anomaly is associated with the highest rate of adverse pregnancy outcomes. Hysteroscopic septoplasty is associated with marked improvement in reproductive outcome in patients with history of recurrent pregnancy loss.

Septate uterus is the term given to complete uterine septum, while subseptate uterus refers to incomplete septum.[1]

Uterine septum should be suspected in patients presenting with:

- Recurrent pregnancy loss
- Infertility
- Bad obstetric history
- Renal anomalies

Objectives

- The aim of this procedure is to divide the uterine septum completely in its mid-portion and to restore the normal morphology of the endometrial cavity.
- Care should be taken to avoid immediate complications, such as uterine perforation or late complication, such as intrauterine scar tissue formation or uterine rupture during pregnancy or delivery.

Indications

- Patients with uterine septum and a complaint of:
  - Recurrent pregnancy loss
  - Infertility
  - Bad obstetric history

Contraindications

- Absolute contraindication:
  - Infection
  - Pregnancy
  - Uterine cancer
- Relative contraindication:
  - Uterine bleeding

Preoperative Assessment

- Hysterosalpingogram (HSG):
  - HSG cannot differentiate between uterine septum and bicornuate uterus.
  - The sensitivity and specificity of HSG in the diagnosis of incomplete uterine septum is poor.[2]
- Transvaginal 2D ultrasound (US), especially with saline sonohysterogram (SIH) in transverse view (endometrial separation in the upper uterine segment).
- Transvaginal 3D US, especially with SIH has led to an increase in the detection rate of such anomalies by allowing visualization in a coronal view.
- MRI should only be ordered if the diagnosis cannot be made by the above tests.
- Diagnostic hysteroscopy is the gold standard to confirm the diagnosis.

Equipment

- Anesthesia personnel and equipment.
- Patient positioning and cervical exposure.
- Video imaging.
- Cervical dilators.
- Hysteroscopic resectoscope.
- Automated fluid management system.

- Uterine distending media (isotonic solutions such as 0.9% normal saline, electrolyte-free solutions such as glycine 1.5%, sorbitol 3%, mannitol 5%).
- The choice of the distension media will depend on whether one uses hysteroscopic bipolar hysteroscopic resectoscope (isotonic solutions such as 0.9% normal saline) or monopolar hysteroscopic resectoscope (electrolyte-free solutions).

Operative Techniques

- All operations should be performed under general anesthesia during the mid-follicular phase of the menstrual cycle or while the patient is on oral contraceptives.
- Cytotec 200 mg is used vaginally the night before the procedure.
- Diagnostic hysteroscopy is usually initially performed to confirm the diagnosis.
- Diagnostic laparoscopy should also be performed:
  - To confirm the diagnosis of a uterine septum, if needed.
  - In infertile patients as part of their work-up.
  - If combined approach is required in difficult cases.
- A 10 mm Gyrus (ACMI) hysteroscopic resectoscope (Division of Olympus; Maple Grove, MN, USA) with a zero degree or 12 degree lens and a straight resectoscope loop is used to resect the septum at 70W cutting and 50 coagulation current with a blend of one setting (authors' preference). This is a monopolar resectoscope requiring electrolyte-free solution as a distension medium.
- The septum should be transected transversely in the midline, avoiding drifting towards the posterior or anterior wall. Such drifting can be avoided by maintaining transection at the plane of both uterine tubal openings.
- When the junction between the septum and myometrium is reached, small arteries may be seen pulsating. If these are cut, they bleed upon division, indicating that the septum has been transected completely.
- With the symmetric visual view of the uterotubal junctions and the laparoscopic uniform translucency of the hysteroscopic light (if concomitant laparoscopy is performed), the operator can safely transect the uterine septum without danger of perforation.[3]
- The procedure is considered complete upon achieving a triangular and symmetrical uterine cavity.
- At the completion of the procedure, the intrauterine pressure produced should be lowered to less than 50 mmHg. This helps in identifying areas of bleeding. Usually, small bleeders stop on their own, but if the number of active arterial bleeders is significant,

these can be individually coagulated with the tip of the electrode.[4]
- Careful and continuous monitoring for any fluid deficit is mandatory.
  - The lowest intrauterine pressure necessary for adequate distension should be used (preferably at a level below the mean arterial pressure). A good range for operative procedures is 70–80 mmHg.
  - Take the necessary steps to terminate the procedure if fluid deficit of electrolyte-free solution is approaching 750–1000 cc.
  - Conclude the procedure if fluid deficit of non-electrolyte solution is 1000–1500 cc of electrolyte-free solution or 2500 cc of normal saline.
  - If fluid deficit of electrolyte-free solution is 1000–1500 cc, order stat electrolytes to rule out hyponatremia and, while waiting for the results, administer one liter of 0.9% normal saline and 10 mg furosemide intravenously.
  - If fluid deficit of electrolyte solution is >2500 cc, order stat electrolytes to rule out hyponatremia and watch for fluid overload. While waiting for the results, administer 10 mg furosemide intravenously and initiate management plan.
  - Serum sodium <120 mmol/L requires critical care setting and a consult with a specialist in critical care medicine.

Postoperative Care

- Postoperative care should include placing a pediatric Foley catheter (size 8 French) inside the endometrial cavity, and inflating its balloon with 3 cc of normal saline for 7 days.
- No need for antibiotics.
- All patients should be placed on estrogen treatment for 6 weeks, adding progestogen during the last 10 days of the estrogen course.
- Postoperative evaluation of the endometrial cavity should be performed 8 weeks after surgery using transvaginal saline SIH with 2D and 3D US.
- Attempts at pregnancy should be postponed for 2 months after surgery because postoperative hysteroscopy with biopsy has shown the uterine cavity to be normal at 8 weeks after surgery.[4]

REFERENCES

1. American Fertility Society, "The American Fertility Society Classifications of Adnexal Adhesions, Distal Tubal Occlusion, Tubal Occlusion Secondary to Tubal Ligation, Tubal Pregnancies, Müllerian Anomalies and Intrauterine Adhesions," *Fertility and Sterility* 49 (1988): 944–55.

2. N. Kallia, O. Abuzeid, M. Ashraf, and M. Abuzeid, "Role of Hysteroscopy in Diagnosis of Subtle Uterine Anomalies in Patients with Normal Hysterosalpingography," *Fertility and Sterility* 96(3)Supplement (2011): S12.

3. M.F.M. Mitwally and M. Abuzeid, "Operative Hysteroscopy for Uterine Septum," in *Textbook of Infertility and Assisted Reproduction*, edited by B.R.M. Rizk, J.A. García-Velasco, H.N. Sallam, and A. Nakrigiannakis, 115–31. Cambridge: Cambridge University Press, 2008.

4. G.B. Candiani, P. Vercellini, L. Fedele, et al. "Repair of the Uterine Cavity After Hysteroscopic Septal Incision." *Fertility and Sterility* 54 (1990): 991.

36

Hysteroscopic Lysis of Intrauterine Adhesions

Bolonduro Oluwamuyiwa and Mostafa Abuzeid

Background and Pathogenesis

Asherman syndrome was first described in 1948 by Joseph Asherman.[1] This syndrome indicates the presence of intrauterine adhesions that obliterate or obstruct the uterine cavity.[1] Any insult severe enough to damage the decidua basalis of the endometrium, leading to granulation tissue formation, can lead to intrauterine synechiae and adherence of the opposing uterine.[2] These adhesions are classically formed following vigorous curettage for the management of incomplete or missed miscarriage (90% of cases), postpartum hemorrhage, or termination of pregnancy. The incidence of adhesions after one abortion is 16.3% and rises to 32% after three or more abortions.[3] Intra-uterine adhesions lead to partial or complete obliteration of the endometrial cavity. Intra-uterine adhesions can be filmy, moderate or dense.

Diagnosis

- Although Asherman syndrome may result in amenorrhea, most women with intrauterine adhesions present with infertility, recurrent pregnancy loss, hypomenorrhea or dysmenorrhea, as opposed to amenorrhea.[1,4]
- The diagnosis of Asherman syndrome is based on a high index of suspicion.
- In women with a suspicious history, failure to have a withdrawal bleed after exogenous estrogen and progesterone treatment may demonstrate end organ endometrial damage and corroborate clinical suspicion.[1]
- When suspected, transvaginal ultrasound scan may demonstrate an element of hematometra at time of menses in patients with partial Asherman syndrome.
- Transvaginal saline infusion sonohysterogram (2D and 3D) and hysterosalpingogram may confirm the presence, location, and extent of intra-uterine adhesions.
- Hysteroscopy, however, is the gold standard for diagnosis.[1]

Management

- As opposed to blind curettage, hysteroscopic lysis of intrauterine adhesions is the primary treatment modality for intrauterine synechiae.[1] It was first performed in 1973.[4]
- Simultaneous laparoscopy or transabdominal ultrasonography may help maintain orientation and thus prevent uterine perforation.[1,3]
- Best results are achieved when central adhesions are lysed first, moving from the lower uterine segment to the fundus, and then to the margins of the cavity, gradually restoring the cavity architecture.[1]
- Sharp dissection, maintenance of distension, and an experienced reproductive surgeon are keys to success.[1,3,4]
- More than one surgical procedure may be required to achieve satisfactory results.
- Best outcomes are achieved in the presence of partial and filmy intra-uterine adhesions.
- Poor prognosis is to be expected in the presence of complete and dense intra-uterine adhesions.

Required Equipment[3]

- Anesthesia personnel and equipment.
- Patient positioning and cervical exposure.
- Video imaging.
- Cervical dilators.
- Operative hysteroscope or hysteroscopic resectoscope.
- Hysteroscopic scissors (flexible or semi-rigid), resectoscope electrodes, Versapoint, Nd-YAG laser, monopolar needle electrode. The instrument to be used is a choice of the operator.
- Bipolar Thermachoice electrode for thick vascularized adhesions.
- Automated fluid management system.

- Uterine distending media (CO_2, isotonic solutions such as 0.9% normal saline, electrolyte-free solutions such as glycine 1.5%, sorbitol 3%, mannitol 5%).

Described Techniques

- Often, thin and fragile synechiae may be lysed by using the tip of the hysteroscope, aided by pressure provided by continuous infusion of the distension media.[1,4]
- Lysis of intra-uterine adhesions using a balloon catheter under fluoroscopic control with local anesthesia or intravenous sedation has been described.[1]
- Thick adhesions may require flexible or better semi-rigid scissors, the resectoscope, electro-dissection, Versapoint or the Nd-YAG laser.[4]
- Laparoscopic injection of leukomethylene blue dye into the uterus to help identifying the junction at which the anterior and posterior walls were attached has been described.[3]
- Choice of distension media will depend on the technique used. Isotonic solutions such as 0.9% normal saline can be used if hysteroscopic scissors or bipolar electrodes are used, while monopolar electrodes require the use of electrolyte-free solutions.
- Careful and continuous monitoring for any fluid deficit is mandatory.
- The lowest intrauterine pressure necessary for adequate distension should be used (preferably at a level below the mean arterial pressure).
- A good range for operative procedures is 70–80 mmHg.
- Take the necessary steps to terminate the procedure if fluid deficit of electrolyte-free solution is approaching 750–1000 cc.
- Conclude the procedure if fluid deficit of non-electrolyte solution is 1000–1500 cc of electrolyte-free solution or 2500 cc of normal saline.
- If fluid deficit of electrolyte-free solution is 1000–1500 cc, order stat electrolytes to rule out hyponatremia, and while waiting for the results, administer one liter of 0.9% normal saline and 10 mg furosemide intravenously.
- If fluid deficit of electrolyte solution is >2500 cc, order stat electrolytes to rule out hyponatremia and watch for fluid overload. While waiting for the results, administer 10 mg furosemide intravenously and initiate management plan.
- Serum sodium <120 mmol/L requires critical care setting and a consult with a specialist in critical care medicine.

Post-Op Management

- Exogenous estrogen (such as Estrace 2 mg orally BID), for 6 weeks after surgery is thought to encourage endometrial re-epithelialization and proliferation. If treatment with a progestin (such as Provera 10 mg daily) in the last 10 days of estrogen course is followed by menses, a return of function is demonstrated.[1]
- Insertion of an intrauterine balloon catheter for 10–14 days after adhesiolysis is thought to keep the uterine walls separated during the healing process, thus decreasing the chance for recurrence.[1]
- Treatment with doxycycline and NSAIDs helps decrease uterine cramping and minimize the risk of infection while the catheter is in place.[1]
- A significant reduction in the formation of adhesions was noted with the postoperative instillation of hyaluronic acid gel following hysteroscopic procedures.[3]
- Surgical results should be assessed after menses by transvaginal saline infusion sonohysterogram (2D and 3D), hysterosalpingogram or "second look" hysteroscopy.[1]

Outcome

- Menstrual function is restored in 52%–88% of cases.[1]
- Reproductive function:
  - The reproductive outcome of women with intrauterine adhesions is generally poor.[5]
  - Following adhesiolysis, the pregnancy outcome is greatly improved.[1]
  - Among women with infertility, live birth rates after hysteroscopic lysis of adhesion range between 25% and 35%.[1]
  - In women who achieve pregnancy, the instances of placenta accreta, placenta previa, preterm birth, and postpartum hemorrhage are higher.[1]
- A high recurrence rate exists, ranging from 20%–60% in severe cases.

REFERENCES

1. M. Fritz and L. Speroff, *Clinical Gynecologic Endocrinology and Infertility*, 8th ed. 459–60, 1175–6, 1204. Philadelphia, PA: Lippincott Williams & Wilkins, 2011.
2. K. Chapman and R. Chapman, "Asherman's Syndrome: A Review of the Literature, and a Husband and Wife's 20-Year World-Wide Experience," *Journal of the Royal Society of Medicine* 83(9) (1990): 576–80.
3. J.A. Rock and H.W Jones, III, *TeLinde's Operative Gynecology*, 10th ed. 336, 355–57, 777. Philadelphia, PA: Lippincott Williams & Wilkins, 2011.
4. J. Berek, *Berek & Novak's Gynecology*, 15th ed. 788–97. Philadelphia, PA: Lippincott Williams & Wilkins, 2012.
5. J.G. Schenker and E.J. Margalioth, "Intrauterine Adhesions: An Updated Appraisal," *Fertility and Sterility* 37(5) (1982): 593–610.

37

Hysteroscopic Management of Submucosal Fibroids

Salem Joseph and Mostafa Abuzeid

Introduction

The presence of a submucosal fibroid may decrease reproductive potential and may be associated with menorrhagia and iron deficiency anemia. Leiomyomas are associated with infertility, with the causal relationship being more evident for submucosal myomas.

Submucosal myomas are associated with recurrent pregnancy loss and obstetric complications, such as premature birth. Submucosal myomas are classified according to the European Society for Hysteroscopy and are divided into three types: Type 0 has no intramural extension, Type I has less than 50% intramural extension and Type II has greater than 50% intramural extension.[1] Hysteroscopic myomectomy has been used successfully in treating submucosal fibroids. This procedure offers better compliance and lower morbidity and costs.[2] Hysteroscopic myomectomy has been shown to be effective in improving fertility and success rates with assisted reproduction.[3]

Indications

- Patients with submucosal fibroids complain of:
  - Infertility
  - Recurrent pregnancy loss
  - Bad obstetrical history
  - Menorrhagia (however, the patients often want to preserve reproductive function or their uterus)

Contraindications of Hysteroscopy

- Absolute
  - Infection
  - Pregnancy
  - Uterine cancer
- Relative
  - Uterine bleeding

Objectives

- The aim of this procedure is to remove the submucosal fibroid completely, preferably in one session, to restore the normal morphology of the endometrial cavity.
- This can usually be achieved in case of Type 0 and some Type I submucosal fibroids.
- Some cases with Type I submucosal fibroids may require more than one session.
- A Type II submucosal fibroid is usually removed laparoscopically or by laparotomy, although it can be removed hysteroscopically by a very experienced operator, usually in more than one session.
- Care should be taken to avoid immediate complications, such as uterine perforation, or late complications, such as intrauterine scar tissue formation or uterine rupture during pregnancy or delivery.

Preoperative Assessment

- Hysterosalpingogram (HSG).
- Transvaginal 2D ultrasound (US) especially with saline sonohysterogram (SIH).
- Transvaginal 3D US, especially with SIH, may help in determining the location and extent of myometrial involvement by allowing visualization in a coronal view.
- MRI may be needed in patients with multiple fibroids.
- Diagnostic hysteroscopy is the gold standard to confirm the diagnosis.
- Concomitant diagnostic laparoscopy may be considered in patients with Type II submucosal fibroid or as part of work-up for infertility.

Equipment

- Anesthesia personnel and equipment.
- Patient positioning and cervical exposure.
- Video imaging.
- Cervical dilators.
- Hysteroscopic resectoscope or hysteroscopic morcellator.
- Automated fluid management system.
- Uterine distending media (isotonic solutions such as 0.9% normal saline, electrolyte-free solutions such as glycine 1.5%, sorbitol 3%, mannitol 5%).
- The choice of the distension media will depend on whether one uses hysteroscopic morcellator or bipolar hysteroscopic resectoscope (isotonic solutions such as 0.9% normal saline) or monopolar hysteroscopic resectoscope (electrolyte-free solutions).

Operative Techniques

- All operations should be performed under general anesthesia during the mid-follicular phase of the menstrual cycle or while the patient is on oral contraceptives.
- Cytotec 200 mg is used vaginally the night before the procedure.
- Diagnostic hysteroscopy is usually initially performed to confirm the diagnosis and type of submucosal myoma.
- Local injection of vasopressin (20 units in 100 cc) in the uterine cervix may reduce excessive bleeding and fluid deficit during the procedure.

Using the Hysteroscopic Resectoscope

- The cervix is progressively dilated to a number 9 Hegar dilator.
- An automated fluid-monitoring system.
- A 10 mm Gyrus (ACMI) hysteroscopic resectoscope (Division of Olympus; Maple Grove, MN, USA) with a zero degree or 12 degree lens and a curved (right angle) resectoscope loop is used to resect the fibroid at 70–100W cutting and 50 coagulation current with a blend of one setting (authors' preference). This is a monopolar resectoscope requiring electrolyte-free solution as a distension medium.
- The myoma is progressively shaved down to the level of the endometrium and until the surface appears to follow the contours of the uterus.
- If a Type I submucosal myoma is removed, the resectoscope could be used to scope the part of the fibroid buried in the myometrium.

- The lowest intrauterine pressure necessary for adequate distension should be used (preferably at a level below the mean arterial pressure).
- A good range for operative procedure is 70–80 mmHg.
- The pieces of the resected myoma are removed using a polyp forceps at the end of the procedure or as needed during the procedure if the view is masked, especially if the myoma is located on the posterior wall.
- The uterine cavity is then assessed for hemostasis and adequacy of resection after stopping infusion of distension medium.
- Careful and continuous monitoring for any fluid deficit is mandatory.
- Take the necessary steps to terminate the procedure if fluid deficit of electrolyte-free solution is approaching 750–1000 cc.
- Conclude the procedure if fluid deficit of non-electrolyte solution is 1000–1500 cc of electrolyte-free solution or 2500 cc of normal saline.
- If fluid deficit of electrolyte-free solution is 1000–1500 cc, order stat electrolytes to rule out hyponatremia and, while waiting for the results, administer one liter of 0.9% normal saline and 10 mg furosemide intravenously.
- If hyponatremia is present, consider stat consult with intensive care specialist to assume management.
- If fluid deficit of electrolyte solution is >2500 cc, order stat electrolytes to rule out hyponatremia and watch for fluid overload. While waiting for the results, administer 10 mg furosemide intravenously and initiate management plan.

Using the Hysteroscopic Morcellator[4]

- Hysteroscopic myomectomy can also be performed using a hysteroscopic morcellator.
- The use of a hysteroscopic morcellator, MyoSure (Hologic) and TRUCLEAR (Smith & Nephew), makes hysteroscopic myomectomy a safer procedure for the gynecologist.
- The use of normal saline as a distension medium reduces the risk of fluid overload.
- The potential for thermal injury is eliminated because these mechanical devices require no electric energy.
- In hysteroscopic morcellation, the resected tissue is contained and delivered through the morcellation system into a collecting pouch.

Postoperative Assessment

- A pediatric Foley catheter (size 10 French) is placed inside the endometrial cavity, and its balloon is inflated with 4 cc of normal saline for 7 days.
- No antibiotic is administered.
- All patients are placed on estrogen treatment (Estrace 2 mg daily) for 6 weeks.
- Progestogen is added during the last 10 days of the estrogen course.
- Postoperative evaluation of the endometrial cavity is performed using transvaginal SIH with 2D and 3D US after 8 weeks.

REFERENCES

1. K. Wamsteker, M.H. Emanuel, and J.H. de Kruif, "Transcervical Hysteroscopic Resection of Submucous Fibroids for Abnormal Uterine Bleeding: Results Regarding the Degree of Intramural Extension," *Obstetrics & Gynecology* 82 (1993): 736–40.
2. N. Makris, E. Vomvolaki, G. Mantzaris, K. Kalmantis, J. Hatzipappas, and A. Antsaklis, "Role of a Bipolar Resectoscope in Subfertile Women with Submucous Myomas and Menstrual Disorders," *Journal of Obstetrics and Gynaecology Research* 33(6) (2007): 849–54.
3. H. Fernandez, O. Sefrioui, C. Virelizier, A. Gervaise, V. Gomel, and R. Frydman, "Hysteroscopic Resection of Submucosal Myomas in Patients with Infertility," *Human Reproduction* 16(7) (2001): 1489–92.
4. T.W.O Hamerlynck, V. Dietz, and B.C. Schoot, "Clinical Implementation of the Hysteroscopic Morcellator for Removal of Intrauterine Myomas and Polyps. A Retrospective Descriptive Study," *Gynecological Surgery* 8 (2011): 193–6.

38

Saline Infusion Sonohysterography

Alan Bolnick and Mostafa Abuzeid

Introduction

Saline infusion sonohysterography (SIS) with transvaginal ultrasound (US), both by 2D and 3D, is a modest outpatient procedure intended to help appraise the endometrial cavity and the endometrium and categorize the uterine cavity silhouette.

Indications

- To evaluate the endometrial cavity in patients presenting with:
  - Infertility.
  - Recurrent pregnancy loss.
  - History of poor obstetrical outcomes.
  - Dysfunctional uterine bleeding.
  - Menometrorrhagia.
- SIS should be performed when the followings pathologies are suspected:
  - Congenital uterine malformations such as T-shaped uterus, unicornuate uterus, bicornuate uterus and uterine septum.
  - Uterine cavity lesions such as uterine fibroids, endometrial polyps, endometrial synechiae.
- SIS should be performed for postoperative assessment following hysteroscopic surgery for uterine septum, submucosal fibroid, endometrial polyps, or hysteroscopic lysis of intrauterine scar tissue.

There are several reasons why transvaginal US may not document structures otherwise detected by SIS. Small abnormalities may not be seen on conventional ultrasonography, because of a collapsed endometrial cavity[1] and when the mass conforms to the shape of the endometrial cavity.[2]

Contraindications

- Suspected pregnancy
- Infection
- Bleeding

Timing of SIS

- This typically is scheduled in the early follicular phase of the menstrual cycle, immediately after cessation of menstrual flow and well before ovulation.
- The endometrium is relatively thin during the early proliferative phase of the cycle, which facilitates imaging interpretation.
- In the late luteal phase of the cycle, thickened endometrium or focal irregularities in the endometrial outline may be misidentified as endometrial hyperplasia or small polyps.
- Alternatively, the procedure can be done while the patient is on oral contraceptive pills.

Technique

- SIS is a very simple process and takes about 5 minutes to complete.
- A pilot transvaginal US is recommended to investigate the uterus and adnexa for any abnormal findings.
- The process must be performed under sterile conditions, since saline may initiate infection into the peritoneal cavity after it passes the genital tract.
- The SIS is started by gently inserting a vaginal speculum (a suitable sized one) into the vagina to visualize the cervix.
- The cervix is cleansed with antiseptic solution.
- A disposable thin flexible catheter is introduced into the cervical canal and the balloon at the catheter tip is placed in the lower uterine segment or cervical canal and 2 cc of air is used to distend the balloon.
- The vaginal speculum is then removed judiciously so as not to disrupt the catheter.
- Subsequently, the transvaginal US probe (preferably 3D) is placed into the vagina and under sonographic guidance, sterile normal saline solution (5–10 mL) is slowly introduced into the endometrial cavity.
- The fluid expands the endometrial cavity, separating the walls, allowing better assessment of the contour

and shape of the endometrium and can demonstrate abnormalities, such as endometrial polyps and intracavitary fibroids.

- Three-dimensional US volume examining can be achieved using a high-resolution three-dimensional US machine.
- When optimal distension of the endometrial cavity is accomplished, a 3-dimensional volume sweep of the sagittal and transverse planes of the uterus can be achieved. Scanned volumes are evaluated in multiplanar 3-dimensions.
- Since the distended balloon may confuse pathology, it is recommended that the balloon be partially deflated immediately before the end of the procedure. The catheter is slowly withdrawn in the cervical canal while adding more fluid to ensure adequate visualization of the lower uterine segment and cervical canal.
- Office analyses of uterine morphology and the endometrial cavity are performed in reconstructed coronal plane.
- The level of pain experienced is usually minimal, with most women experiencing either no pain or only mild cramping period-type discomfort during the test.
- It is suggested taking 2 NSAID tablets 30–60 minutes before the procedure to mitigate any discomfort.
- No anesthesia is required.
- The patient can eat and drink normally before and after the procedure.
- Prophylactic antibiotics are not administered, unless there is a history of chronic pelvic inflammation.

Complications

- SIS is a very innocuous procedure with minimal post-procedure complaints, including cramping, spotting, and vaginal discharge.
- One serious complication that has been observed is pelvic infection, occurring less than 1% of the time and can be seen in women with a history of pelvic inflammatory disorder.

Diagnostic Characteristics Seen by SIS

- Endometrial polyps emerge as solitary or multiple, diffuse or focal, sessile or pedunculated.
- Polyps are isoechoic compared to the endometrium.
- An endometrial polyp may occur either alone, in the setting of endometrial hyperplasia, or less commonly, as carcinoma.[3]
- The position of a submucosal leiomyoma can be detected through SIS by its echogenicity and the percentage of the myoma that protrudes into the uterine cavity.[4]

- Myomas are hypo- to isoechoic in relation to the myometrium.
- Endometrial hyperplasia may be assumed sonographically. The principal findings are a thickness of >15 mm or >8 mm and the presence of a non-homogenous echo pattern with microcystic changes.
- With SIS, adhesions are typically seen as echogenic, mobile strands of tissue that intersect the endometrial cavity, attaching to both uterine walls.[4]

Comparison of SIS to Other Diagnostic Modalities

- The sensitivity and specificity of transvaginal US, SIS, and diagnostic hysteroscopy in detecting intracavitary abnormalities were 56.3%, 72%, 81.3% and 100%, 87.5%, 100%, respectively.
- SIS is very effective for evaluating uterine myomas and was comparable to hysteroscopy in detecting submucosal myomas (and determining their intramural component) and locating other intramural myomas.[5]
- SIS is a safe and highly sensitive and specific method in the diagnosis of endometrial polyps. Its results closely correspond to those obtained in a hysteroscopic examination and histopathological analysis.
- Three dimensional SIS is highly accurate in the diagnosis of uterine cavity abnormalities such as uterine septum. SIS has the potential to eliminate unnecessary hysteroscopic surgery.

REFERENCES

1. S. Laifer-Narin, N. Ragavendra, E.K. Parmenter, and E.G. Grant, "False-Normal Appearance of the Endometrium on Conventional Transvaginal Sonography: Comparison with Saline Hysterosonography," *American Journal of Roentgenology* 178(1) (2002): 129–33.
2. E. Moschos, R. Ashfaq, D.D. McIntire, B. Liriano, and D.M. Twickler, "Saline-Infusion Sonography Endometrial Sampling Compared with Endometrial Biopsy in Diagnosing Endometrial Pathology," *Obstetrics and Gynecology* 113(4) (2009): 881–7.
3. A. Shushan, A. Revel, and N. Rojansky, "How Often Are Endometrial Polyps Malignant?" *Gynecologic and Obstetric Investigation* 58(4) (2004): 212–15.
4. F.P. Leone, D. Timmerman, T. Bourne, et al., "Terms, Definitions and Measurements to Describe the Sonographic Features of the Endometrium and Intrauterine Lesions: A Consensus Opinion from the International Endometrial Tumor Analysis (IETA) Group," *Ultrasound in Obstetrics & Gynecology* 35(1) (2010): 103–12.
5. S. Kelekci, E. Kaya, M. Alan, Y. Alan, U. Bilge, and L. Mollamahmutoglu, "Comparison of Transvaginal Sonography, Saline Infusion Sonography, and Office Hysteroscopy in Reproductive-Aged Women with or Without Abnormal Uterine Bleeding," *Fertility and Sterility* 84(3) (2005): 682–6.

39

General Principles of Laparoscopy

Rubin Raju and Mostafa Abuzeid

Contraindications[1]

Absolute

- Lack of surgical skills or equipped operating room
- Contraindications to Trendelenburg positioning (retinal detachment, raised intracranial pressure, etc.)
- Shock

Relative

- Advanced pregnancy
- Hemodynamic instability
- Large abdominopelvic mass suspicious for malignancy
- Ventriculo-peritoneal shunts

Required Equipment

- Straight catheter/Foley catheter
- Weighted vaginal speculum
- Deaver's retractor
- Single-toothed tenaculum
- Uterine manipulator (Cohen cannula, ACORN, HUMI or Sponge-stick)
- Scalpel and blade
- Allis or Kocher clamps, towel clips
- Laparoscopic setup: camera, light source, fiber-optic cord, insufflator and tubing
- Laparoscope-0°; 5 mm or 10 mm
- Veress needle
- Trocar and sleeves—5 mm or 10 mm
- Argon beam coagulator (Birtcher Medical System, Irvine, CA, USA)
- Standard laparoscopy tray set
- Laparoscopic instruments (needle driver, scissors, graspers—depending on the planned surgery)
- 4-0 Vicryl sutures or skin glue

Preparation on the Day prior to Surgery

- Ask patient to remain NPO overnight or at least 8 hours prior to surgery, depending on anesthesia protocol.
- Patient may take certain home medications with a sip of water on the morning of surgery.
- Medical clearance, if needed.
- Perform a urine pregnancy test.

Patient Preparation and Positioning

- The anesthesiologist administers general anesthesia.
- Place patient in lithotomy position using stirrups.
- Make sure buttocks are at edge of table or slightly over the edge. Make sure that the thigh is flexed ≤90 degrees and hips are abducted ≤45 degrees, to avoid nerve injury.[2]
- Position arms securely on the sides of the patient, with padding.
- Perform standard "time out" identifying patient and procedure.
- Perform vaginal prep using Betadine prep or non-iodine-based prep in iodine-allergic patients.
- Perform an abdominal skin and perineal skin iodine based/Betadine prep. Use non-iodine-based prep in iodine-allergic patients.
- Drape patient in a sterile manner.
- Perform an examination under anesthesia.
- Empty bladder using a straight catheter/Foley catheter.
- Place weighted speculum on posterior vaginal wall.
- Use a Deaver's retractor to retract the anterior vaginal wall.
- Grasp anterior lip of cervix with single-toothed tenaculum.
- Place the uterine manipulator into the cervix and then remove the weighted speculum.

- Lower legs to achieve a low lithotomy position, with the patient's thighs 160°–170° to the abdomen.
- Remove top glove or change gloves.
- Turn attention to abdomen and prepare for performing laparoscopy.

Surgical Setup[2]

- A right-handed surgeon usually should stand on the patient's left side with the assistant on the patient's right.
- Place the video monitors per the surgeon's and assistant's visual convenience, commonly near the patient's lower legs. If only one video monitor is present, place it between the patient's legs.
- Place the insufflation monitor across the surgeon so that the intra-abdominal pressure can be viewed.
- Place all the tubing and cords away from the surgical field and secure them to the drapes.

Choosing Initial Trocar Entry[1]

- Decide where to place initial trocar: umbilicus (commonly), above umbilicus, or Palmer's point. Use Palmer's point (1–2 cm inferior to left costal margin in mid-clavicular line) in patients with a midline scar or when extensive abdominal/pelvic adhesions are suspected. For Palmer's point, ask anesthesiologist to place nasogastric tube to decompress the stomach. Make a 5 mm or 10 mm sub-umbilical transverse or longitudinal skin incision with a number 11 size scalpel blade when using umbilical approach.
- Dissect incision with a hemostat up to fascia.

Abdominal Entry[1,2]

Decide whether to use open or closed (Veress needle, direct trocar with or without the camera) technique.

Open Technique[1]

- Grasp fascia with Allis clamps or Kocher clamps and incise fascia vertically about 5–10 mm with scalpel.
- Tag the cut margins of fascia with sutures.
- Insert 5–10 mm Hasson trocar and start insufflation.
- Secure Hasson's trocar to previously placed suture tags.

Closed Technique with Veress Needle[1]

- Elevate abdomen with towel clips applied to edge of umbilicus, or if not, with your hands.

- Introduce Veress needle through incision site into abdominal cavity at 90° angle in an obese patient or at 45° in a thin patient.
- Connect Veress needle to insufflator tubing at low flow (1 L/min).
- Confirm intra-abdominal placement with feeling for double click on insertion, saline drop test, syringe barrel test, aspiration and/or low starting pressure (<10 mmHg).

Closed Technique with Direct Trocar Insertion[2]

- Elevate abdomen as described above.
- Introduce trocar with or without camera through incision site into abdominal cavity at 90° angle in an obese patient or at 45° in a thin patient.
- Remove trocar and replace it with lens and camera.
- Connect sleeve to insufflator tubing at low flow (1 L/min).
- Confirm intra-abdominal placement as described earlier.

Obtaining Pneumoperitoneum[1]

- After confirming intraperitoneal placement, turn CO_2 gas to high flow (>6 L/min) to achieve set intra-abdominal pressure limit of 15 mmHg.
- If Veress needle technique used, remove it and replace it with a 5 or 10 mm trocar, either with or without camera, while elevating the abdominal wall as described above.
- Percuss right hypochondrium to note absence of liver dullness.

Choosing Additional Port Sites[1]

- Place a second port under direct camera vision, commonly two finger breadths above symphysis pubis in midline.
- Remove trocar and replace it with a blunt probe to aid in inspection of pelvic or abdominal cavity.
- Place patient in Trendelenburg position to help move the bowel away from pelvic cavity.
- The location and need for additional port sites should depend on ease of access to pathology.

Closing Port Sites

- Close port sites >10 mm with Carter Thomason or EndoClose closure system, by directly identifying and approximating fascial margins using a 0 Vicryl suture, or by tying fascia suture tags if placed earlier.[1]
- Close skin incisions with 4-0 Vicryl/Monocryl suture or by using skin glue.

REFERENCES

1. T. Bardawil and A. Hernandez-Rey, *Operative Laparoscopy* (2013) http://emedicine.medscape.com/article/1848486-overview#a01.

2. H.T. Sharp, S.L. Francis, and A. Alvarez Murphy, "Diagnostic and Operative Laparoscopy", in J.A. Rock and H.W. Jones, III, *Te Linde's Operative Gynecology*, 10th ed. 325–7. Philadelphia, PA: Lippincott Williams & Wilkins, 2011.

40

Microlaparoscopy

Oscar D. Almeida, Jr.

Required Equipment

- Microlaparoscope: 2 mm fiber-optic microlaparoscope with 50,000 fiber image bundle and a 75° field of view
- Cameras and accessory equipment
  - Zoom lens technology
  - Automatic insufflator
    - CO_2
  - Number 11 scalpel blade
- Microinstrumentation (all 2 mm except for Veress needle)
  - Trocars
    - Veress needle
  - Probe marked in centimeters to assist in measuring fallopian tube length
  - Irrigation/aspiration cannulas
  - Injection/aspiration needle cannulas
  - Forceps
  - Scissors
    - Non-cautery
    - Monopolar cautery
  - Bipolar forceps
  - Endoloops

Accessory Equipment

- Uterine manipulator
  - Insufflation syringe (10 cc)
  - Chromotubation syringe (50–60 cc)
  - Methylene blue dye or indigo carmine dye

Anesthesia/Analgesia

- General
- Conscious sedation
- Local anesthesia

Sample Protocol for Conscious Sedation in Microlaparoscopy

Note: Continuous careful monitoring of the patient, especially the respirator rate, cannot be overemphasized.

- Atropine: 0.2 mg administered preoperatively to reduce the risk of a vasovagal reaction
- Ondansetron hydrochloride: 4 mg to prevent nausea/vomiting
- Midazolam hydrochloride: 1–2 mg, very rarely 3 mg in an obese patient
- Fentanyl citrate: 250 micrograms administered slowly over 10 minutes, and titrated in 50 microgram increments to effect patient comfort
- Prophylactic antibiotic of choice
- 1% lidocaine with epinephrine 1:100,000, 10 mL buffered with sodium bicarbonate 10:1 dilution to decrease tissue irritation

Microlaparoscopic Procedure

- Patient selection
- Thorough physical examination and laboratory work-up
- Informed consent
- "Time out" with the entire surgical team present

Preparing and Monitoring the Patient

- Patient fasting a minimum of 7 hours.
- Intravenous line with Ringer's lactate solution.
- Oxygen via nasal cannula.
- Monitoring includes the use of a continuous ECG, heart rate, and respiratory monitors, pulseoximeter, and automated blood pressure cuff. Data obtained should be charted every 5 minutes.
- Position the patient in the dorso-lithotomy position on operating table.

- Skin is sterilely prepared and draped.
- Consider a Foley catheter.

Microlaparoscopic Procedure

Under General Anesthesia

- Proceed as routine laparoscopy

Under Local Anesthesia with Conscious Sedation

- Administer conscious sedation.
- Application of local anesthetic block to umbilicus.
- Insert Veress needle with the 2-mm trocar and insufflate CO_2. **Note:** Better patient tolerance of procedure if CO_2 insufflation is under 1.5 L.
- Close incisions with Dermabond.

Conditions Evaluated with Diagnostic Microlaparoscopy and Limited Operative Microlaparoscopy under Local Anesthesia with Conscious Sedation

The applicability of this approach is that many procedures done as traditional laparoscopy under general anesthesia may be performed in a more minimally invasive manner.

- Diagnosing pelvic inflammatory disease
- Diagnosing hemorrhagic ovarian cysts
- Evaluating right lower quadrant pain (acute appendicitis; other chronic abnormalities of the appendix)
- Evaluating infertility (chromotubation)
- Evaluation of pelvic pain (conscious pain mapping)
- Diagnosing and, in select cases, lysis of adhesions
- Diagnosis of endometriosis (visually and via biopsy) and, in select cases, fulguration of endometriosis
- Ovarian drilling
- Monitor ectopic pregnancy being treated with methotrexate

BIBLIOGRAPHY

Almeida, O.D. Jr. (ed). *Microlaparoscopy*. New York: Wiley-Liss, 2000.

Almeida, O.D. Jr. "Microlaparoscopy in the Evaluation of Infertility: New Horizons." In *Clinical Infertility and In Vitro Fertilization*, edited by B. Rizk and H. Sallam. New Delhi: Jaypee, 2012.

Almeida, O.D. Jr. and B. Rizk. 1998. "Microlaparoscopic Ovarian Drilling Under Local Anesthesia." *Middle East Fertility Society Journal* 3: 189–91.

41

Laparoscopic Myomectomy and Mini-Laparotomy: An Alternative Approach for Myomectomy

Ahmed Abdelaziz and Mostafa Abuzeid

Introduction

Myomectomy is advisable for women who wish to preserve their childbearing capabilities.[1] In this regard, minimally invasive surgery has been shown to be a valid alternative to the standard open technique. The Da Vinci robotic assisted laparoscopic myomectomy has been used shown to be the most successful and easy to learn minimally invasive approach.[2] However, robotic surgery is expensive, and not available in many parts of the world. In addition, the recent non-availability of an automatic morcellator has created challenges with respect to morcellation of large fibroids.[3]

Meanwhile laparoscopic myomectomy has several disadvantages. Experienced laparoscopic surgeons can only perform it after a long learning curve. The technical difficulty of laparoscopic suturing and the smaller number of sutures used to close the uterine defect may lead to a hematoma formation within the myometrium. This may lead to infection and a weak uterine scar. Some of these problems can be overcome be using continuous running suture with V-lock (Covidien, Mansfield, MA, USA). Excessive use of electrocautery may result in more tissue damage that may weaken the uterine scar. There have even been some case reports of uterine rupture after laparoscopic myomectomy.[4] Therefore the need for an alternative approach that is less invasive than standard laparotomy is increasingly desirable. To overcome these problems, mini-laparotomy during laparoscopic myomectomy is used to overcome the challenges standing against laparoscopic myomectomy, while preserving the advantage of minimally invasive surgery.[5]

Indications of Mini-Laparotomy During Laparoscopic Myomectomy

- Large myoma (≥8 cm)
- Large/deep defect in the myometrium
- Multiple myomas
- Vascular myoma (to reduce blood loss)

- Entry of the endometrial cavity during myomectomy to reduce intrauterine scar tissue formation by adequate repair of endometrial cavity

Preoperative Assessment

- CBC with type and screen
- 2D and 3D transvaginal ultrasound scan (US)
- 2D and 3D transvaginal saline infusion sonohysterogram (SIH)
- 2D transabdominal US and/or MRI in patients with large or multiple uterine fibroids

Operative Technique

- Normal entry of the abdomen using any of the techniques described in the literature for laparoscopy.
- Four surgi-ports should be used, one sub-umbilical, one supra-pubic, and two additional surgi-ports should be placed lateral to inferior epigastric vessels, one on each side.
- Exploring the abdomen and identifying any abnormality.
- Confirming the diagnosis of fibroid and assessing the number, site and size of the fibroid.
- Tubal perfusion to determine tubal patency.
- Attention directed towards the fibroid, where diluted Pitressin (20 iu in 100 cc of saline) is injected in the area of the myometrium where the fibroid is attached to the uterus.
- With a laparoscopic spatula connected to a monopolar cautery (30W cutting current and 30W coagulation current and a blend of one setting), a transverse incision is made in the serosa, cutting down to the myometrium until the fibroid capsule is reached.

- A 5 or a 10 mm laparoscopic myomectomy single-toothed grasper is used to grasp the fibroid and it is dissected in steps from the uterine wall.
- Coagulation of any blood supply to the fibroid using spatula connected to monopolar cautery in order to reduce blood loss, during dissection of the fibroid.
- Evaluating the entrance of the endometrial cavity is done by injecting diluted indigo carmine dye transcervically and observing for any dye in the myoma bed.
- A 5 cm transverse skin incision is made in the suprapubic region; the skin is dissected in an upward and downward fashion to allow a longitudinal incision in the fascia.
- The rectus muscle is separated in the midline and the peritoneum is entered in routine fashion.
- The uterus is lifted up partially through the mini-laparotomy incision using a uterine manipulator to facilitate suturing. This allows better visualization of the myometrial defect.
- The defect in the myometrium is repaired using 2-0 Vicryl sutures either with interrupted figure of eight sutures or in continuous running fashion.
- The serosal layer is repaired with 3-0 Vicryl sutures using a baseball running suture.
- The myoma is brought up through the small incision and is morcellated using a scalpel.
- Fascia and skin are closed in layers.
- Foley catheter (10 French) is placed into the uterine cavity and the balloon is inflated with 4–5 cc of normal saline to reduce intrauterine scar tissue formation in cases in which the endometrial cavity is entered. The Foley catheter is left for 7 days.
- In such cases, the patient is placed on estrogen tablets (such as Estrace 2 mg/day) for 6 weeks, starting on postoperative day 3. Progestogen (such as Provera 10 mg) is added during the last 10 days of the estrogen course to facilitate endometrial healing).
- Patient is discharged home the next day.

Postoperative Assessment

- Patients are instructed not to get pregnant for at least 3 months.
- Endometrial cavity is assessed post-operatively using transvaginal US (2D and 3D) with SIH if the endometrial cavity was entered.
- The mode of delivery should be by cesearean section if the endometrial cavity was entered.

REFERENCES

1. P.C. Klatsky, N.D. Tran, A.B. Caughey, and V.Y. Fujimoto, "Fibroids and Reproductive Outcomes: A Systematic Literature Review From Conception to Delivery," *Obstetrics & Gynecology* 198 (2008): 357.
2. J. Pundir, V. Pundir, R. Walavalkar, K. Omanwa, G. Lancaster, and S. Kayani, "Robotic-Assisted Laparoscopic Vs Abdominal and Laparoscopic Myomectomy: Systematic Review and Meta-Analysis," *Journal of Minimally Invasive Gynecology* 20 (2013): 335–45.
3. D. Larraín, B. Rabischong, C.K. Khoo, R. Botchorishvili, M. Canis, and G. Mage, "Iatrogenic Parasitic Myomas: Unusual Late Complication of Laparoscopic Morcellation Procedures," *Journal of Minimally Invasive Gynecology* 17 (2010): 719–24.
4. G. Pistofidis, E. Makrakis, P. Balinakos, E. Dimitriou, N. Bardis, and V. Anaf, "Report of 7 Uterine Rupture Cases After Laparoscopic Myomectomy: Update of the Literature," *Journal of Minimally Invasive Gynecology* 19 (2012): 762–74.
5. R. Singh, S. Joseph, M. Ashraf, and M. Abuzeid, "Laparoscopic Myomectomy Followed by Minilaparotomy for Management of a Large Submucous Fibroid," *Journal of Gynecologic Surgery* 29(3) (2013): 161–4.

42

Laparoscopic Excision of a Large Endometrioma

Rubin Raju and Mostafa Abuzeid

Introduction

Endometriosis is the presence of endometrial glands and stroma outside the uterus; endometriomas are cysts formed by the presence of deep-seated endometriosis in the ovary. They indicate an advance stage of endometriosis.

Required Equipment and Materials

- Video laparoscopy equipment
- Standard diagnostic and operative laparoscopy tray set
- Additional laparoscopic instruments:
  - 5 mm laparoscopic Teflon probe (Elmed Chicago, IL, USA)
  - 5 mm atraumatic grasper × 2 (Wolf, Vernon Hills, IL, USA)
  - 5 mm toothed grasper
  - 5 mm needle driver with pointed tip (Wolf, Vernon Hills, IL, USA)
  - 5 mm monopolar diathermy needle tip (Elmed, Chicago, IL, USA)
  - Argon beam coagulator (Birtcher Medical System, Irvine, CA, USA)
  - CO_2 laser (OmniGuide Surgical, Cambridge, MA, USA)
- Seprafilm (Genzyme Corporation, Cambridge, MA, USA)
- Adept (Baxter, Deerfield, IL, USA)
- Floseal (Baxter Healthcare Corporation, Hayward, CA, USA)

Patient Preparation prior to Surgery

- Determine ovarian reserve by antral follicle count (AFC), AMH, and day 2–3 FSH and LH levels as patients with large endometrioma may have an element of diminished ovarian reserve and excision of

an endometrioma may lead to further diminished ovarian reserve.[1]
- Order a CA-125 level. Other tumor markers determine if other pathologies are considered in the differential diagnosis of the ovarian cyst.
- Transvaginal ultrasound scan to evaluate the number and sizes of the endometriomas.
- Transvaginal ultrasound scan is also performed to determine the presence of hydrosalpinx, which is commonly present in patients with endometrioma.
- Counsel the patient regarding the possibility of oophorectomy during surgery and the possibility of diminished ovarian reserve after surgery.

Techniques of Excision/Ablation of Endometriomas[2,3]

- Endometriomas <1 cm are opened, evacuated, and the lining is ablated with the argon beam coagulator or CO_2 laser.
- Endometriomas >1 cm are managed with excision of the cyst wall.
- Endometriomas can be excised intact, but most likely they will burst during ovariolysis or dissection of the endometrioma.
- If needed, perform adhesiolysis to achieve full mobilization of the ovary using blunt dissection or with the use of laparoscopic scissors. Often the cyst ruptures during this step.
- A longitudinal incision is then carefully made on the cortex overlying the cyst, generally along the antimesenteric border on the opposite side to the hilum.
- If the cyst ruptures, immediately drain the contents with a suction cannula and irrigate the cavity and the pelvic cavity. Avoid spread of the chocolate materials in the upper abdomen.
- The site of rupture is then extended using a monopolar diathermy needle tip.
- Inspect the cavity for suspicious features like papillary structures.

- Determine the plane of dissection between the ovarian cortex and the cyst wall by zooming on the area. Sometimes scissors are used to cut a small part of ovarian and cyst wall tissues to allow visualization of the plane of cleavage, especially in areas of thin ovarian cortical tissue.

- The normal ovarian tissue is stabilized with two atraumatic graspers.

- The cyst wall is grasped with a toothed grasper and stripped gently from the bed of the normal ovarian tissue. Avoid pulling the toothed grasper away from the ovarian tissue. Instead, stripping should be by pulling gently in a downward direction.

- Any remaining fragments of the cyst wall that were still adhered to the ovarian bed are coagulated with the argon beam coagulator (40W with 2 L flow rate) or vaporized CO_2 laser (8–10W in a continuous mode).

- The argon beam coagulator or CO_2 laser (defocused beam) is also used to coagulate any bleeding points on the ovarian bed. Occasionally, Floseal can be used if there is bleeding from the hilum that is not controlled by pressure with a 4×4 gauze for a few minutes.

- Most authorities leave the defect in the ovarian cortex to heal spontaneously.

- The authors of this chapter prefer to close the defect; therefore, ovarian cortex reconstruction is performed with one or two interrupted vertical mattress sutures using 4-0 Vicryl.

Reducing Postoperative Adhesion Formation

- To reduce adhesion formation, place an adhesion barrier like Seprafilm slurry (three 3×6 inch sheets made into a slurry by dissolving in 60 cc of normal saline) on the ovarian cortex.

- Alternatively, adhesion barrier solutions like Adept (500–700 cc) can also be placed into the peritoneal cavity.

- Temporary ovarian suspension may be performed for advanced endometriosis in an attempt to reduce the risk of recurrence of adhesions between ovarian fossa and ovaries.[4]

Surgical Management of Concomitant Endometriosis

- Argon beam coagulation can be used to coagulate or the CO_2 laser to vaporize suspicious spots of endometriosis found anywhere in the pelvis.

- If endometriosis is found on the pelvic sidewall near the ureter, on the bladder or bowels, use argon beam coagulator or CO_2 laser with extra care to avoid injury to such vital organs.

- If peritubal adhesions are present, perform salpingolysis using Teflon probe and micro-diathermy needle using laparoscopic microsurgical principals.[5]

- If fimbrial phimosis or hydrosalpinges is found, perform fimbrioplasty or salpingostomy or salpingectomy as indicated.[5]

Postoperative Follow-Up

- AMH and FSH levels after 2 months
- Transvaginal ultrasound scan

REFERENCES

1. E. Somigliana, N. Berlanda, L. Benaglia, et al., "Surgical Excision of Endometriomas and Ovarian Reserve: A Systematic Review on Serum Antimüllerian Hormone Level Modifications," *Fertility and Sterility* 98 (2012): 1531.

2. M.I. Abuzeid, A. Ahmed, K. Sakhel, R. Alwan, M. Ashraf, M. Mitwally, and M. Diamond, "Unilateral Versus Bilateral Adnexal Disease in Stage III and Stage IV Endometriosis Does Not Affect Pregnancy Outcome After Operative Laparoscopy," *Obstetrical & Gynecological Survey* 64(7) (2009): 452–3.

3. J.S. Hesla and J.A. Rock, "Endometriosis", in J.A. Rock and H.W. Jones, III, *Te Linde's Operative Gynecology*, 10th ed. 457–9. Philadelphia, PA: Lippincott Williams & Wilkins, 2011.

4. M.I. Abuzeid, M. Ashraf, and F.N. Shamma, "Temporary Ovarian Suspension at Laparoscopy for Prevention of Adhesions," *Journal of American Association Gynecologic Laparoscopy* 9(1) (2002): 98–102.

5. M. Mitwally, A. Thotakura, O. Abuzeid, M. Ashraf, M. Diamond, and M.I. Abuzeid, "Suturing Versus Flowering Technique of Bruhat After Fimbrioplasty for Endometriosis-Related Infertility," *Gynecological Surgery* 6(2) (2009): 147–52.

43

Laparoscopic Management of Subtle Fimbrial Pathology Secondary to Endometriosis

Omar Abuzeid and Mostafa Abuzeid

Background

The presence of subtle fimbrial pathology in infertile women with early stages of endometriosis has been documented.[1] Three types of fimbrial pathology were identified:

- Fimbrial agglutination: One or more adhesive bridges of fimbria across the ostium.
- Fimbrial blunting: Fimbrial adherence side by side.
- Fimbrial phimosis: Actual narrowing of the fimbriated end.

Some patients with fimbrial phimosis have a concentric stricture of the fallopian tube at its distal end noted at the ampullary fimbrial junction. During tubal perfusion in these patients, there is dilation of the distal ampullary portion of the fallopian tube, and the dye is spilled out as a narrow stream. Other subtle pathologies near the fimbriated end of the fallopian tube include:

- Accessory ostium and diverticulum.[2]
- Paratubal cyst near the fimbriated end of the tube.[2]

Diagnosis

- The initial workup for tubal pathology before surgery should include: history and physical, family history of endometriosis, sexual history, history of sexually transmitted diseases (STDs), pelvic inflammatory disease, previous surgical and medical history, as well as any other infertility history.
- The patient should undergo a thorough work-up, including:
  - Transvaginal ultrasound scan to determine the presence of possible endometrioma, adenomyosis, and hydrosalpinx.
  - Hysterosalpingogram may suggest the presence of subtle fimbrial pathology when there is minimal spillage of the dye or by the presence of localized dye around the distal ends of the tubes.
- Diagnostic laparoscopy is the only way to confirm the diagnosis of subtle fimbrial pathology. Thus, it should preferably be performed by a surgeon who has experience not only in identifying distal fimbrial pathology, but also in performing laparoscopic tubal surgery.
- The techniques used to assess the fimbria depend not only on inspection by zooming towards and gently grasping the fimbria with an atraumatic grasping forceps, but also on the use of a Teflon probe while injecting diluted indigo carmine. Also the fimbriated end of the tube should be assessed by underwater examination.

Required Equipment and Materials

- Video laparoscopy equipment
- Standard diagnostic and operative laparoscopy tray set
- Additional laparoscopic instruments:
  - 5 mm monopolar diathermy needle tip (Elmed, Chicago, IL, USA)
  - 5 mm laparoscopic Teflon probe (Elmed Chicago, IL, USA)
  - 5 mm atraumatic grasper × 2 (Wolf, Vernon Hills, IL, USA)
  - Argon beam coagulator (Birtcher Medical System, Irvine, CA, USA)
- CO_2 laser (OmniGuide Surgical, Cambridge, MA, USA)

Techniques of Laparoscopic Surgical Correction (Fimbrioplasty)

- Fimbrial agglutination: Deglutination is performed by lifting the fimbrial bands using laparoscopic Teflon Probe, then these bands are divided using monopolar diathermy needle tip (cutting current of 20W).

- Fimbrial phimosis, prefimbrial phimosis, and fimbrial blunting: Fimbrioplasty procedure is performed by incising the antimesenteric side (1–1.5 cm length) using monopolar needle tip cautery while probing the fimbrial end by a Teflon probe.

- In order to keep the new fimbrial ostium adequately opened, the edges of the fimbrial ostium should be everted by the technique of heating the serosal surfaces of the tube around the fimbrial ostium using the argon beam coagulator (flowering technique of Bruhat).[3,4]

- All through the procedure, irrigation and suction should be performed using heparinized Lactated Ringer's solution (5000 IU in 1 liter).

- Argon beam coagulator can be used to coagulate or CO_2 laser to vaporize suspicious spots of endometriosis found anywhere in the pelvis.

REFERENCES

1. M. Abuzeid, M. Mitwally, A. Ahmed, E. Formentini, M. Ashraf, O. Abuzeid, and M. Diamond, "The Prevalence of Fimbrial Pathology in Patients with Early Stages of Endometriosis," *Journal of Minimally Invasive Gynecology* 14 (2007): 49–53.
2. M. Ashraf and M.I. Abuzeid, "Subtle Distal Tubal Pathology," in G.N. Allahbadia, E. Saridogan, O. Djahanbakhch, and R. Merchant, *The Fallopian Tube*, 458–66. Tunbridge Wells: Anshan, 2009.
3. M. Canis, G. Mage, J.L. Pouly, H. Manhes, A. Wattiez, and M.A. Bruhat, "Laparoscopic Distal Tuboplasty: Report of 87 Cases and a 4-Year Experience," *Fertility and Sterility* 56 (1991): 616–21.
4. M.F.M. Mitwally, A. Thotakura, M. Ashraf, O. Abuzeid, M.P. Diamond, and M. Abuzeid, "Suturing Versus Flowering Technique of Bruhat after Fimbrioplasty for Endometriosis-related Infertility," *Gynecological Surgery* 6(2) (2009): 147.

44

Laparoscopic Management of Mature Cystic Teratoma

Rahima Sanya and Mostafa Abuzeid

Introduction

Teratomas have 15%–25% incidence.[1] They represent 20%–40% of ovarian neoplasms,[1] and are the most common ovarian neoplasm encountered in surgery. The average age of presentation is 20–30 years; it is bilateral in 10%–15%.[1]

Pathogenesis

- Derived from all three layers: ectoderm (skin), mesoderm (muscle, fat), and endoderm: (epithelium-thyroid, gastrointestinal, etc.).[2]
- Slow growing.
- Tumor arises from a single germ cell after the first meiotic division.[2]
- Pathology: unilocular cyst with sebaceous material, lined by squamous epithelium. Can contain hair, mucous, bone and other tissue.[1]

Diagnosis

- Ultrasound shows a cyst with the most common findings:[1]
  - Rokitansky nodule (usually contains bone and teeth).
  - Echogenic mass, usually hair with sebaceous material.
  - Multiple thin echogenic bands, representing hair.
  - Fluid levels due to sebaceous fluid floating on top of the cyst fluid.
- Ultrasound has 98% PPV, 85% sensitivity.[1]

Clinical Presentation/Complications

- Asymptomatic (50%)—incidental finding during pelvic exam.[1]

- Rarely: thyroid storm due to thyroid tissue known as struma ovarii.
- Present with ovarian torsion (10%), strong association once tumor >11 cm.[1]
  - Will present with abdominal pain, nausea or vomiting, or hemodynamic instability.
  - Is a clinical diagnosis.
  - Ultrasound has a diagnostic accuracy of 74.6%.[3]
  - O/E: An adnexal mass usually anterior to uterus because of its fat content making it float.
- Cyst rupture: 1% causing granulomatous peritonitis.[1]
- 1%–2% malignant degeneration especially at age 60–70s.[1]

Required Equipment and Materials

- Video laparoscopy equipment
- Standard diagnostic and operative laparoscopy tray set
- Additional laparoscopic instruments:
  - 5 mm laparoscopic Teflon probe (Elmed Chicago, IL, USA)
  - 5 mm atraumatic grasper × 2 (Wolf, Vernon Hills, IL, USA)
  - 5 mm toothed grasper
  - 5 mm needle driver with pointed tip (Wolf, Vernon Hills, IL, USA)
  - 5 mm monopolar diathermy needle tip (Elmed, Chicago, IL, USA)
- Argon beam coagulator (Birtcher Medical System, Irvine, CA, USA) or CO_2 Laser Seprafilm (Genzyme Corporation, Cambridge, MA, USA), Flow seal
- 5000 U of heparin in 1 L Lactated Ringer for irrigation

Patient Preparation prior to Surgery

- Transvaginal ultrasound scan.
- CBC.
- Prepare patient for possible oophorectomy and salpingectomy, if irreversible damage to tube and ovary, or patient does not desire fertility.

Technique of Cystectomy with Sparing of Ovarian Tissue

- De-torsion—watch for reperfusion of ovary and fallopian tube, try to mobilize ovary to give time for assessing the reperfusion.
- Assess size of cyst: laparoscopy for large cysts has high risk of rupture vs. laparotomy.
- If needed, adhesiolysis should be done with laparoscopic scissors to mobilize ovary.
- A longitudinal incision is then made on the ovarian cortex covering the cyst, preferably at the antimesentery border (away from hilum of ovary) using a monopolar needle tip.
- If the cyst ruptures, copious suction and irrigation of the contents should be performed throughout the abdomen. Otherwise suction contents of cyst by inserting probe into incision.
- The incision site is then extended using monopolar diathermy needle tip.
- Find a cleavage plane between ovarian cortex and cyst; sometimes extending the incision may enhance visualization.
- The normal ovarian tissue is stabilized with two atraumatic graspers.
- Grasp cyst wall with toothed grasper and strip gently from ovarian cortex using traction in a downward motion and counter-traction with the atraumatic graspers.
- Remaining cortex is then coagulated with the argon beam coagulator (40W with 2 L flow rate) or vaporized CO_2 laser (8–10W in a continuous mode) to obtain hemostasis.
- If bleeding is seen at the hilum: use Floseal.
- Ovarian cortex defect can be left open or closed; we prefer closing the defect using interrupted mattress sutures. Starting with the deep space, lateral wall of ovary is approximated with 4–0 Vicryl.
- Use an Ethicon Endobag to scoop the residual cyst tissue and to remove it from port.
- Always inspect the other ovary.

Reducing Postoperative Adhesion Formation

- To reduce adhesion formation, place an adhesion barrier on the ovarian cortex.
- Lactated Ringer irrigation approximately 1 L left in the abdomen.

Future Management

- One study showed in pediatric and adolescent populations following ovarian cystectomy, 3% will recur.[4]
- Adult population recurrence: 0%–7.6% depending on type of surgery for cystectomy.[5]
- Annual ultrasound—literature does not suggest specific frequency.

REFERENCES

1. E.K. Outwater, E.S. Siegelman, and J.L. Hunt, "Ovarian Teratomas: Tumor Types and Imaging Characteristics," *Radiographics* 21 (2001): 475.
2. D. Linder, B. Kaiser McCaw, and F. Hecht, "Parthenogenic Origin of Benign Ovarian Teratomas," *New England Journal of Medicine* 292 (1975): 63–6. DOI: 10.1056/NEJM197501092920202.
3. R. Mashiach, N. Melamed, N. Gilad, G. Ben-Shitrit, and I. Meizner, "Sonographic Diagnosis of Ovarian Torsion: Accuracy and Predictive Factors," *Journal of Ultrasound in Medicine* 30(9) (2011): 1205–10.
4. E.M. Rogers, L. Allen, and S. Kives, "The Recurrence Rate of Ovarian Dermoid Cysts in Pediatric and Adolescent Girls," *Journal of Pediatric and Adolescent Gynecology* 27(4) (2014): 222–6.
5. P.Y. Laberge and S. Levesque, "Short-Term Morbidity and Long-Term Recurrence Rate of Ovarian Dermoid Cysts Treated by Laparoscopy Versus Laparotomy," *Journal of Obstetrics and Gynaecology Canada* 28(9) (2006): 789–93.

45

Tubal Cannulation for Proximal Tubal Disease

Wael Salem, Osama A.H. Abu Zinadah, Joshua Ekladios, and Botros Rizk

Introduction

Tubal surgery was the sole treatment modality for women experiencing tubal factor infertility until the widespread use of assisted reproductive technologies (ART) in the 1980s. With the ongoing improvements in ART, tubal surgery for tubal factor infertility became less popular among clinicians and patients alike. Despite this general trend, the outcomes for tubal surgery yield good results and are particularly advantageous for young women who have no other etiologies for their infertility. In actuality, tubal surgery and ART complement each other and the decision to attempt one approach over the other should be based on the anticipated chance of success, the patient's risk factors, cost-effectiveness and the patient's reproductive goals.

Epidemiology and Etiology

- Tubal disease accounts for approximately 25%–35% of female infertility, with proximal tubal blockage comprising up to 10%–25% of cases of tubal occlusion.
- The etiology for tubal blockage can be attributed to pelvic inflammatory disease (PID) in up to 50% of cases and generally affects the tube at multiple sites.
- The remaining 50% of tubal blockage are mostly due to endometriosis, salpingitis isthmica nodosa, and obstructing lesions in the uterine cavity.

Tubal Cannulation

- Tubal cannulation is a minimally invasive technique to treat proximal intratubal blockage.
- There are a variety of uses for intratubal catheterization.
- The following conditions were noted to respond to tubal catheterization: tubal spasm, cornual polyps amorphous debris, stromal edema, mucosal agglutination, chronic salpingitis, endometriosis, salpingitis isthmica nodosa and intrauterine synechiae.

- While these etiologies could be addressed with tubal cannulation, the diagnosis is not necessarily evident in many cases and a thorough history and diagnostic evaluation should guide treatment.

Diagnostics

- Patients undergoing an evaluation for tubal patency will most often receive a hysterosalpingogram (HSG).
- It is advantageous as it is a minimally invasive outpatient procedure.
- However, it is limited by a false positive rate that can be as high as 50%.
- The gold standard for tubal evaluation is laparoscopy with chromopertubation.
- This is often indicated if there is a high suspicion for pelvic conditions, such as PID or endometriosis.
- In conjunction with a routine infertility evaluation and a thorough history, the patient can then be risk-stratified to assess whether tubal cannulation offers a reasonable chance of success to address the underlying tubal blockage.

Technique

- Tubal cannulation has been demonstrated to allow re-cannulation of up to 85% of obstructed tubes with a subsequent 30% rate of re-occlusion.
- After proper patient selection, the patient should undergo a routine preoperative evaluation for operative hysteroscopy and laparoscopy.
- A diagnostic laparoscopy to precede the hysteroscopic portion of the case allows for a more thorough evaluation of the pelvis and possibly the site of tubal occlusion.
- It also offers the benefit of chromopertubation to follow hysteroscopy in order to photographically document tubal patency.

- A diagnostic hysteroscopy should be done with the intention of identifying any intrauterine pathology with particular attention to any pathology that may interfere with the tubo-cornual junction.

Procedure

- After assembly of the tubal cannulation system (Modified Novy Cornual Cannulation set, Cook Ob/Gyn, IN, USA) a 5 mm hysteroscope is introduced into the uterine cavity with the introducing catheter and obturator in place.
- Identification of both tubal ostia should aid in creating an operative plan.
- Next, the 5-French catheter and obturator are advanced in unison through the operative channel and advanced into the ostium and proximal tube.
- The obturator is then removed.
- The guide wire is advanced to the level of the outer catheter.
- A 3-French inner catheter is subsequently introduced over the guide wire through the tubal ostium.
- Care should be taken at this point to interpret the amount of tactile feedback on the guidewire. An increased intratubal pressure and decreased compliance portend a poor prognosis.
- The procedure is then to be repeated on the contralateral side.
- Chromopertubation may be done unilaterally or bilaterally.

Postoperative Course and Follow-Up

- As this is an outpatient procedure, it is generally very well tolerated.
- Though rare, possible adverse effects may include tubal dissection, tubal perforation, or damage to an otherwise normal tube.
- It is unclear if the recannulation procedure itself leads to higher rates of ectopic pregnancy.

Conclusion

Pregnancy rates following tubal cannulation range from 12%–57%. Ultimately, one of the most important aspects of tubal cannulation is to correctly identify the correct patient candidate. In young women with bilateral proximal tubal occlusion and no other causes for infertility, consideration of tubal cannulation as a first line treatment before *in vitro* fertilization offers many benefits, including a natural pregnancy process, decreased costs, avoidance of IVF-related complications, and the possibility for subsequent pregnancies.

BIBLIOGRAPHY

Capitanio, L., A. Ferraiolo, S. Croce, et al. 1991. "Transcervical selective salpingography: a diagnostic and therapeutic approach to cases of proximal tubal injection failure." *Fertility and Sterility* 55: 1045–50.

Confino, A., I. Tur-Kaspa, A. De Cherney, et al. 1990. "Transcervical balloon tuboplasty. A multicentre study." *Journal of American Medical Association* 264: 2079–82.

Das, K., T. Nagel, and J. Malo. 1995. "Hysteroscopic Cannulation for Proximal Tubal Obstruction: A Change for the Better?" *Fertility and Sterility* 63: 1009–15.

Das, S., L.G. Nardo, and M.W. Seif. 2007. "Proximal Tubal Disease: The Place for Tubal Cannulation." *Reproductive BioMedicine Online* 15(4): 383–8.

Gleicher, N. and V. Karande. 1996. "The Diagnosis and Treatment of Proximal Tubal Disease." *Human Reproduction* 11(9): 1823–8.

Novy, M.J. 1995. "Transhysteroscopic Techniques For Tubal Catheterization." *Références en Gynécologie Obstétrique* 67–71.

Novy, M., A.S. Thurmond, P. Patton et al. 1988. "Diagnosis of Cornual Obstruction by Transcervical Fallopian Tube Cannulation." *Fertility and Sterility* 50: 434–40.

46

Robotic Assisted Laparoscopic Myomectomy

Hashem Lotfy, Arsany Bassily, Lauren Mann, and Botros Rizk

Introduction

Uterine myomas are the most common tumor of the female genital tract, affecting 20%–50% of women of reproductive age. Uterine myomas can present with a variety of clinical symptoms, depending on the size, site, and number of myomas. These presentations may include abnormal uterine bleeding, infertility, recurrent pregnancy losses, dysmenorrhea, and pressure symptoms. Myomectomy is the surgical option of choice for women who desire to preserve their uterus.

Myomectomy

Myomectomy can be done via laparotomy, laparoscopy, or robotic assisted laparoscopy.

- Performing myomectomy through laparotomy carries the disadvantages of longer hospital stay, longer recovery time, increased blood loss, and more liability to the formation of intra-abdominal adhesions.
- On the other hand, the technical difficulties of enucleation of some myomas that may not be accessible to most laparoscopic surgeons and the lack of the precision that is required for meticulous multilayered closure of the myoma bed limit the use of laparoscopy in myomectomy.
- Robotic surgery has the advantages of being a minimally invasive surgery with small abdominal incisions, less blood loss, and shorter hospital stay. In addition, it offers the surgeon free motion of the laparoscopic arms in a way that mimics the human hand, rather than the limited movements of the arms of the traditional laparoscopy. This major advantage, together with the magnified 3D image of the surgical field, allows the surgeon to perform myomectomies that are difficult to do by laparoscopy alone.

Equipment

- Da Vinci robot consists of three parts:
  - Surgeon console: The surgeon console is composed of a binocular stereoscopic vision system that transmits the image from an endoscope of diameter 12 mm in Da Vinci Si or 8 mm in the Da Vinci Xi robot, which contains two 5 mm diameter cameras which generate the 3D image of the surgical field. The surgeon's hand movements are transmitted to control the arms and the camera via two handles which are also capable of abolishing fine tremors. The surgeon can also use his/her foot to control several pedals used for cautery (unipolar, bipolar, ultrasound), moving the camera, and for repositioning of the instruments and interchange the arms.
  - Patient side trolley: The Da Vinci S, Si and Xi robots come with four arms: one arm holds the camera and the other three arms hold different instruments used during the procedure. The arms of the robot are equipped with (Endowrist) joints which allow free motion of the arms in all directions.
  - Imaging system: The vision system is composed of an insufflator, a light source, and a dual camera.
- Hysteroscopic removal device (Myosure (Hologic), TRUCLEAR (Smith & Nephew), or Sympthion, Boston Scientific).
- Uterine manipulator.

Technique

- General anesthesia is induced.
- Patient is seated in lithotomy position.

- Hysteroscopy should be done for diagnosis of associated endometrial hyperplasia, uterine polyps, or submucosal fibroids.
- Hysteroscopic tissue removal device (Myosure (Hologic), TRUCLEAR (Smith & Nephew), or Symphion, Boston Scientific) can be used as a diagnostic tool and to remove submucosal myomas.
- A uterine manipulator is inserted within the uterine cavity.
- A 12 mm camera (8 mm camera in Da Vinci Xi) is inserted in the midline at the level of the umbilicus or above according to the size of the uterus.
- Visualization of the peritoneal cavity and assessment of the size, site, and accessibility of the myomas in addition to peritoneal adhesions.
- Two 8 mm robotic trocars are placed under visualization 10 cm on each side of the midline.
- A forth incision is made in the right upper quadrant for a 12 mm trocar that can be used by the assistant or in the left upper quadrant for the fourth robotic arm.
- Chromotubation is done to ensure tubal patency.
- Pitressin can be injected around myomas to minimize blood loss.
- Uterine incisions are made using monopolar diathermy according to the site and size of myomas.
- Identification of the capsule of compressed uterine wall, then enucleation of myomas inside the avascular plane using traction and counter-traction with the aid of the assistant or the fourth robotic arm.
- Control of bleeding from the uterine wound using the diathermy.
- Suturing of the myoma bed in layers using absorbable Vicryl 0 or V-Loc.
- Extraction of myomas:
  - Small and medium-sized myomas can be cut using the scissors and then extracted.
  - In March 2014 the FDA banned the use of morcellators due to accusations that it caused dissemination and upstaging of leiomyosarcoma.
  - Since then, a number of alternative solutions have been suggested to extract large myomas out of the human body.
  - A mini-laparotomy or morcellation of myomas inside protective bags can be done.

Limitations

- The lack of tactile sensation may lead to missing some intramural myomas, which can be overcome with an intraoperative ultrasound detecting the location of myomas. Some surgeons prefer a preoperative MRI for accurate detection of the myoma sites.
- Another limitation is the risk of dissemination of tissues into the peritoneal cavity during morcellation of myomas and the possibility of spreading leiomyosarcoma. A safe and feasible method for tissue extraction should be addressed in a way that keeps the advantages of minimally invasive surgery.
- Myomectomy should be reserved for women of reproductive age and should not be performed in postmenopausal women.

BIBLIOGRAPHY

Barakat E.E., M.A. Bedaiwy, S. Zimberg, et al. 2011. "Robotic Assisted, Laparoscopic and Abdominal Myomectomy: A Comparison of Surgical Outcomes." *Obstetrics & Gynecology* 117: 256–65.

Hanafi M.M. and S.C. Garbich. 2011. "Comparative Studies Between Robotic Laparoscopic Myomectomy and Abdominal Myomectomy." *Fertility and Sterility.* 96(3): 167–8.

Nezhat C., O. Lavie, S. Hsu, et al. 2009. "Robotic Assisted Laparoscopic Myomectomy Compared with Standard Laparoscopic Myomectomy: A Retrospective Matched Control Study." *Fertility and Sterility* 91: 556–9.

Pundir J., V. Pundir, R. Walavalker, et al. 2013. "Robotic Assisted Laparoscopic Vs Laparoscopic Myomectomy: Systemic Review and Meta-Analysis." *Journal of Minimally Invasive Gynecology* 20(3): 335–45.

47

Robotic Assisted Tubal Anastomosis after Tubal Sterilization

Hashem Lotfy, Rola Turki, and Botros Rizk

Introduction

Tubal sterilization represents a significant proportion of the methods used for contraception. Although introduced to the patients as an irreversible contraceptive method, many patients ask for restoration of their fertility after having their tubes ligated. For those patients, IVF or surgical tubal reanastomosis are the only available options. Microsurgical tubal reanastomosis can be done by laparotomy or laparoscopy. Laparotomy is accompanied by a high success rate, but it carries the disadvantages of longer hospital stay, increased pain and wound care. A laparoscopic approach overcomes the disadvantages of open surgery, but on the other hand it requires a skilled surgeon, and the learning curve is slow. Robotic surgery led to a revolution in the field of minimally invasive gynecology. It carries the advantages of both open and laparoscopic surgery.

Equipment

- Da Vinci robot consists of three parts:
  - Surgeon console: The surgeon console is composed of a binocular stereoscopic vision system that transmits the image from the endoscope with 12 mm diameter in the Si or 8 mm in the Xi robots, which contains two 5 mm diameter cameras which generate the 3D image of the surgical field. The surgeon's hand movements are transmitted to control the arms and the camera via two handles which are also capable of abolishing fine tremors. The surgeon can also use his/her feet to control several pedals for cautery (unipolar, bipolar, ultrasound), moving the camera, and for repositioning the instruments and to interchange the arms.
  - Patient side trolley: The newer versions of the Da Vinci robot come with four arms: one arm holds the camera and the other three arms hold different instruments used during the procedure. The arms of the robot are equipped with (Endowrist) joints which allow free motion of the arms in all directions.
  - Vision system: The vision system is composed of an insufflator, a light source, and a dual camera.

Procedure

- General anesthesia is induced.
- The patient is placed in lithotomy position.
- A uterine cannula is inserted inside the uterus for both uterine manipulation and chromotubation.
- The 12 mm camera port (8 mm port in Da Vinci Xi robot) is introduced through the umbilicus.
- Two lateral 8 mm ports are placed 10 cm lateral to the midline.
- An accessory 10 mm port is placed on the right upper quadrant to be used for suction irrigation, entry, and removal of suture materials.
- The site of the previous sterilization is divided using the scissors.
- The proximal part of the tube is mobilized, then its end is transected using the scissors.
- The patency of the proximal part is checked via chromotubation.
- The medial end of the distal part of the tube is transected, and its patency is checked using a pediatric feeding tube.
- The mesosalpinx is approximated using one or two interrupted 6-0 polyglactin sutures.
- The mucosa of the tube is then sutured with four interrupted 7-0 sutures, after which the patency of the whole tube is rechecked again by chromotubation.
- Finally, the serosa of the tube is sutured.

Follow-Up

HSG can be done to confirm patency after 3–6 months.

Conclusion

Robotic surgery offers an alternative solution to IVF for women who wish to get pregnant after tubal sterilization. Robotic surgery carries the advantages of laparoscopic surgery, such as decreased blood loss, shorter hospital stay, and faster recovery period. In addition, its rapid learning curve leads to a progressive decrease in the operative time. Robots have been used for tubal reanastamosis after tubal sterilization. The magnified 3D image and the free motion of the laparoscopic arms help surgeons to perform precise suturing of the tubes, which can result in improving the success rates of such a microsurgical procedure.

BIBLIOGRAPHY

Chen, C.C. and T. Falcone. 2009. "Robotic Gynecologic Surgery: Past, Present and Future." *Clinical Obstetrics and Gynecology* 52(3): 335–43.

Dharia-Patel, S.P., M.P. Steinkampf, S.J. Whitten, and B.A. Malizia. 2008. "Robotic Tubal Anastomosis: Surgical Technique and Cost Effectiveness." *Fertility and Sterility* 90(4): 1175–9.

Falcone, T., J.M. Goldberg, H. Margossian, and L. Stevens. 2000. "Robotic Assisted Laparoscopic Microsurgical Tubal Anastmosis: A Human Pilot Study." *Fertility and Sterility* 73(5): 1040–2.

Gardner, D.K., B. Rizk, and T. Falcone (eds). *Human Assisted Reproductive Technology: Future Trends in Laboratory and Clinical Practice*. Cambridge: Cambridge University Press, 2011.

Gordts, S., R. Campo, P. Puttemans, and S. Gordts. 2009. "Clinical Factors Determining Pregnancy Outcome After Microsurgical Tubal Reanastomosis." *Fertility and Sterility* 92: 1198–202.

The Practice Committee of the American Society of Reproductive Medicine. 2015. "Role of Tubal Surgery in the Era of Assisted Reproductive Technology: A Committee Opinion." *Fertility and Sterility* 103(6): 37–43.

48

Unexplained Infertility

Hassan N. Sallam

Definition

There is no universally accepted definition of unexplained infertility. However, the general working definition is couples with unexplained infertility after one year of cohabitation with the following characteristics:

- Proper ovulation and adequate luteinization as shown by a midluteal plasma progesterone concentration of >10 ng/mL.
- At least two normal seminal fluid analyses based on the minimal WHO criteria: a count of 15 million spermatozoa/mL, an initial motility of 40%, a progressive motility of 32%, a vitality of 58%, and a normal (strict) morphology of 4%.
- Patent and properly functioning tubes as shown by both a hysterosalpingogram and a properly performed laparoscopy stating clearly the condition of the fimbria and excluding the presence of endometriosis.
- A normal uterine cavity as shown by hysterosalpingography and hysteroscopy, and an endometrial biopsy showing no granulomata and adequate luteinization.

Possible Causes of Unexplained Infertility

Unfortunately, the diagnosis of unexplained infertility is sometimes applied to couples who were inadequately investigated. Consequently, in these patients, a meticulous search for the following possible causes must be made before embarking on treatment:

The Postcoital Test (PCT)

- The PCT is performed in the immediate pre-ovulatory period 8 to 24 hours (not 2 to 3 hours) after intercourse as it is meant to evaluate the reservoir function of the cervical mucus.
- The mucus is taken from the cervical canal using a tuberculin syringe or similar device.

- A positive test shows good ovulatory-type mucus containing a good number of progressively motile spermatozoa.

Luteal Phase Defect

- The mere observation of signs of ovulation on ultrasonography does not necessarily mean that adequate luteinization has taken place. Thus, a luteal phase defect may still be present.
- The condition has traditionally been diagnosed on the basis of endometrial histology.
- However, the measurement of mid-luteal plasma progesterone is a more practical and reliable index and the calculation of the mean of three readings taken on days 19, 21 and 23 of the menstrual cycle is an even more reliable method. The mean mid-luteal plasma progesterone concentration in cycles resulting in a full term singleton pregnancy was 25 ng/mL, with pregnancy not continuing if the level is less than 10 ng/mL.
- Alternatively, the area under the curve of plasma progesterone, during the whole of the luteal phase, can be calculated.

Luteinized Unruptured Follicle (LUF) Syndrome (also called Trapped Ovum Syndrome)

- In this condition, the ovum is not extruded from the follicle despite the presence of all systemic manifestations of ovulation.
- The exact cause remains unclear.
- The condition is associated with luteal phase insufficiency and poor endometrial development.

Minimal Endometriosis

- Minimal endometriosis (clear vesicles, pink vascular lesions, white scarred lesions, red lesions, yellow-brown patches and peritoneal windows) is sometimes missed if this is not looked for carefully during diagnostic laparoscopy.

TABLE 48.1

Step 1.
Controlled ovarian
  hyperstimulation and intrauterine
  insemination (COH + IUI)
	• This treatment will overcome: any luteal phase defect, the presence of luteinized unruptured follicles, any undiagnosed minimal endometriosis, and a doubtful PCT.
	• If pregnancy does not occur after three cycles of therapy, assisted conception is proper.

Step 2.
Combined in vitro fertilization and
  intracytoplasmic sperm injection
  (IVF + ICSI).
	• This treatment will clarify and overcome: the possibility of defective oocytes, sperm defects, and cases of surprising failed fertilization.
	• Half the oocytes are subjected to IVF in order to evaluate the fertilizing capacity of the sperm.
	• The other half are subjected to ICSI to guarantee the presence of embryos for transfer.
	• If failure of fertilization is diagnosed, ICSI should be repeated until pregnancy occurs.
	• Repeated failures of implantation, despite the presence of good-quality embryos, denote the presence of an endometrial factor and prednisolone (5 mg BID starting on day 2 of the cycle) can be added.

• It may be better observed by near-contact laparoscopy, which magnifies the peritoneal area or by "painting" the peritoneum and broad ligament with blood or serosanguinous fluid to render atypical lesions more evident.

Failed Fertilization

• Many couples with unexplained infertility show repeated failure of fertilization at IVF despite the presence of good-looking oocytes and spermatozoa. This failure of fertilization may be due to sperm defects which cannot be detected in the classical semen analysis or to poor quality of the oocytes.

• Regardless of the cause of failed fertilization, intracytoplasmic sperm injection (ICSI) is the logical treatment in these cases as it can bypass any faulty mechanisms in the spermatozoa or oocytes responsible for this problem.

Uterine Factor

• Unexplained infertility may be due to gross abnormalities of the uterus or due to intrauterine lesions (uterine septum, fibroids, endometrial polyps, or intrauterine synechiae).

• These abnormalities can be diagnosed on hysterosalpingography and by performing a meticulous hysteroscopic examination of the uterine cavity.

Defective Implantation

• Proper implantation of the embryo is the result of an interplay between the TH2 reaction (favoring implantation by producing blocking antibodies and mediated through IL-4, IL-5, IL-6, IL-9, IL-10 and IL-13) and the TH1 reaction (favoring rejection by producing natural killer cells and mediated through IFN-γ, IL-2, IL-12 and TNF-α).

• Conditions favoring the TH1 reaction over the TH2 reaction may lead to repeated early pregnancy loss or to failure of implantation of the embryo.

Management of Unexplained Infertility

Numerous treatment modalities have been suggested for those who remain infertile, including controlled ovarian hyperstimulation (COH), intrauterine insemination (IUI), gamete intrafallopian transfer, IVF, ICSI, or any combination of these. Based on the current literature, the scheme in Table 48.1 is suggested.

BIBLIOGRAPHY

Aboulghar, M.A., R.T. Mansour, G.I. Serour, M.A. Sattar, and Y.M. Amin. 1996. "Intracytoplasmic Sperm Injection and Conventional in Vitro Fertilization for Sibling Oocytes in Cases of Unexplained Infertility and Borderline Semen." *Journal of Assisted Reproduction and Genetics* 13(1): 38–42.

Aboulghar, M.A., R.T. Mansour, and G.I. Serour, et al. 1999. "Management of Long-Standing Unexplained Infertility: A Prospective Study." *American Journal of Obstetrics & Gynecology* 181: 371.

Aboulghar, M., R. Mansour, G. Serour, A. Abdrazek, Y. Amin, and C. Rhodes. 2001. "Controlled Ovarian Hyperstimulation and Intrauterine Insemination for Treatment of Unexplained Infertility Should Be Limited to a Maximum of Three Trials." *Fertility and Sterility* 75(1): 88–91.

Guzick, D.S., M.W. Sullivan, G.D. Adamson, et al. 1998. "Efficacy of Treatment for Unexplained Infertility." *Fertility and Sterility* 70: 207.

Hull, M.G., P.E. Savage, and D.R. Bromham. 1982. "Prognostic Value of the Postcoital Test: Prospective Study Based on Time-Specific Conception Rates." *British Journal of Obstetrics & Gynaecology* 89: 299–305.

Pandian, Z., A. Gibreel, and S. Bhattacharya. 2012. "In Vitro Fertilization for Unexplained Subfertility." *Cochrane Database of Systematic Reviews* 4: CD003357.

Sallam, H.N., A.N. Sallam, F. Ezzeldin, et al. 1999. "Reference Values for Midluteal Plasma Progesterone—Evidence From HMG-Pregnancy Cycles." *Fertility and Sterility* 71: 711.

Sallam, H.N., A.N. Sallam, F.E. Ezzeldin, A.F. Agamia, and A.H. Abou-Ali. 2000. "Minimal Requirements for a Successful Outcome in Anovulatory Patients Treated with Human Menopausal Gonadotropins." *The International Journal of Fertility and Women's Medicine* 45(4): 285–91.

49

Male Evaluation for Infertility

Kiranpreet Khurana, Edmund Sabanegh, Jr., and Ashok Agarwal

Male Evaluation for Infertility

To Be Prepared before Clinic

- Retrieve records from prior evaluation, if any.
- Note pertinent information.

Evaluation in the Clinic—History

- Determine whether infertility is primary (no prior conceptions with any partner) or secondary (if secondary, same partner or different partner).
- Determine how long the couple has been trying to achieve pregnancy.
- Ask if any prediction kits used, ask about coital habits, and frequency of intercourse.
- Inquire about gonadotoxins: lubricants, infections, drugs (medications or illegal), exposures (hyperthermia, cigarette smoking, chemicals, heavy metals), recent illnesses or trauma.
- Assess sexual function (libido, erection, orgasm, ejaculation).
- Any prior evaluation or treatment of infertility or sexual disorders.
- Assess for symptoms of systemic or hormonal diseases (gynecomastia, hot flashes, galactorrhea, loss of libido, facial or body hair loss, abdominal masses, thyroid masses).
- Ask about female partner's age, history of infertility, and any pertinent medical or surgical history. Refer to an obstetrician for further evaluation, if needed.[1]
- Assess patient's other medical and surgical history—diabetes mellitus, cystic fibrosis, prior orchitis, cirrhosis, thyroid dysfunction, varicocele, prostatitis, prior trauma, or inguinal, testicular, or retroperitoneal surgery.
- Assess family history, social history, medications, allergies, and review of systems.

Evaluation in the Clinic—Physical

- Examine genitalia and note Tanner stage.
- Examine penis (presence of lesions, masses, plaques).
- Examine urethral meatus for stenosis, location.
- Examine testicles for size, masses, consistency.
- Examine presence or absence of vas deferens and any palpable defects.
- Examine epididymis and presence of any fullness, cysts (spermatoceles).
- Assess spermatic cord for presence of varicocele.
- Examine prostate for any tenderness and palpably enlarged midline structures.
- Examine rest of body for presence of secondary sexual characteristics, neurological deficits, abdominal masses, skin lesions, thyroid enlargement or masses.

Classification of Male Infertility

After history and physical exam, check semen analysis twice. Can consider basic endocrine tests to include AM testosterone, follicle-stimulating hormone (FSH), and luteinizing hormone (LH) if symptoms of possible endocrinopathy (decreased libido, erectile dysfunction) or abnormal physical exam (gynecomastia, reduced testicular volume) exist.[2]

Based on above evaluation, categorize type of infertility into one of three: pre-testicular, testicular, or post-testicular.[3]

Pre-Testicular Infertility

- Symptoms depend on etiology. Decreased libido and erectile dysfunction most common. May have small testicles on physical exam.
- Testosterone is low; LH and FSH are either low or normal.
- Evaluate for causes: high prolactin (due to prolactinoma, stress, hypothyroidism, renal failure, excess estrogen), pituitary or hypothalamic problem (tumor, trauma, surgery, hemochromatosis,

Kallman's syndrome, Prader–Willi syndrome, Laurence–Moon–Bardet–Biedl syndrome), medications like opioids, exogenous androgens, LHRH agonists, GnRH antagonists.

- If low testosterone, and low or normal LH and FSH, check for above causes by assessing prolactin, TSH, free T4, iron, TIBC, ferritin, and obtain pituitary ± brain MRI with and without gadolinium.

Testicular Infertility

- Symptoms depend on etiology. Decreased libido and erectile dysfunction most common. May have small testicles on physical exam.
- Testosterone is low; LH and FSH are high.
- Evaluate for causes: primary testicular failure, Klinefelter's syndrome, Sertoli cell-only syndrome, maturation arrest, genetic anomalies, structural sperm defects, gonadotoxin exposure, infection, varicocele, cryptorchidism, testicular atrophy, torsion, or absence.
- If low testosterone, high LH and FSH, and semen analysis shows severe oligospermia or azoospermia, offer karyotype and Y chromosome microdeletion analysis as well as genetic counseling.

Post-testicular Infertility

- Symptoms are minimal unless the patient has vasal obstruction due to cystic fibrosis, Kartagener's syndrome, Young's syndrome, or lower urinary tract obstruction due to a stricture. Usually have normal sized testicles, and normal FSH. May have low-volume ejaculate.
- Evaluate for causes: ejaculatory duct obstruction, epididymal obstruction, vasal obstruction or agenesis, vasectomy, anejaculation or retrograde ejaculation, urethral stricture.
- If vas deferens absent on examination, do CFTR mutation testing, genetic counseling, and renal ultrasound.
- If low-volume ejaculate and vas deferens present, check post-ejaculate urinalysis for retrograde ejaculation; if no sperm seen in urinalysis, consider transrectal ultrasound to evaluate for ejaculatory duct obstruction.
- If normal volume ejaculate, may have obstruction in proximal portion of vas deferens or epididymis.

REFERENCES

1. J.T. Choy and P. Ellsworth, "Overview of Current Approaches to the Evaluation and Management of Male Infertility," *Urologic Nursing* 32(6) (2012): 286–94, 304 quiz 295.
2. A. Jungwirth, A. Giwercman, H. Tournaye, et al., "European Association of Urology Guidelines on Male Infertility: The 2012 Update," *European Urology* 62(2) (2012): 324–32.
3. P.J. Stahl, D.S. Stember, and M. Goldstein, "Contemporary Management of Male Infertility," *Annual Review of Medicine* 63 (2012): 525–40.

50

Hysterosalpingography

Islam Fahmi, Mostafa Abuzeid, and Shawky Z.A. Badawy

Introduction

Hysterosalpingogram (HSG) is a simple, safe and relatively inexpensive procedure used to assess the cervical canal, the uterine cavity, and fallopian tubes using X-ray imaging.

Indications

- Suspected congenital uterine malformations
- Suspected uterine cavity lesions
- Suspected tubal lesions
- Postoperative assessment following
  - Hysteroscopic removal of uterine septum, submuosal fibroid, endometrial polyp or hysteroscopic lysis of intrauterine synechae
  - Tubal surgery, lysis of fimbrial agglutination, and salpingostomy
  - Hysteroscopic sterilization surgery (Essure)

Contraindications

- Pregnancy
- Infection (if the patient is at high risk of infection, then prophylactic antibiotics should be used, i.e., doxcycline 100 mg BID for 7 days starting the day before the procedure)
- (Active) bleeding
- Allergy to iodine or any component of the contrast material (in such cases consider sonohysterosalpingography or laparoscopy and hysteroscopy)

Timing of the Procedure

- The patient calls the office on day 1 of her menstrual cycle.
- She is then scheduled in the proliferative phase of her cycle, preferably few day after end of menses or while the patient is on birth control pills.

Patient Preparation

- 1–2 hours before the procedure ibuprofen 600 mg (or equivalent for pain control)
- If the patient is allergic to the contrast:
  - 13 hours before the procedure: prednisone 50 mg
  - 1 hour before the procedure: diphenhydramine 50 mg
  - An IV line should be in place

Instruments

- Radiology suite equipped with fluoroscopy and monitors
- Sterile gloves
- Drape
- Lubricating gel
- Speculum
- Large swab(s)
- Antiseptic solution
- A thin, flexible catheter with a balloon at the end (disposable HSG catheter)
- Single-toothed tenaculum and Kahn (or Rubin) cannula (for difficult cases)
- Sponge forceps
- 20 cc syringe with a 17 gauge needle
- Water-soluble contrast material solution
- Gauze

Contrast Material

- No significant difference in pregnancy rate between water-soluble or oil-soluble.
- Water-soluble contrast has been found to:
  - Be better tolerated.
  - Be quicker on elimination.
  - Provide better detail.

- Oil-soluble contrast has been shown to be associated with granuloma formation and higher allergic reaction rate.
- Following HSG there was no significant difference in pregnancy rate between oil-soluble and water-soluble contrast material.

Technique

- Appropriate identification of the patient.
- Patient empties her bladder.
- Patient placed in the dorsal lithotomy position on the table and draped appropriately.
- The external genitalia cleansed with antiseptic solution.
- A bimanual exam is performed to estimate the size and position of the uterus.
- While wearing sterile gloves and using lubricating gel, insert speculum into the vagina.
- Using a large swab, the cervix is adequately cleansed with antiseptic solution.
- Tenaculum grasps anterior lip of cervix, if required.
- A disposable HSG catheter pre-filled with the radio-opaque dye is introduced through the cervical canal into the lower uterine segment and the balloon is distended with 2 cc of air.
- The speculum is removed and an initial film is taken.
- A scot film is obtained.
- Under fluoroscopy, contrast is injected slowly to minimize the possibility of uterine and/or cornual spasm, and to avoid obscuring subtle filling defects that may not be visible if the contrast is injected rapidly.
- To further minimize the possibility of spasm, the contrast maybe pre-warmed close to body temperature.
- Another film is taken as the contrast starts to fill the uterine cavity.
- Another film is taken when the uterine cavity is filled with contrast to evaluate the uterine cavity as a whole. Sometimes the patient may need to be repositioned at different angles to provide the best visualization.
- As the contrast spills from the uterine cavity into the tubes it is closely observed. The flow pattern of the contrast through the tubes is evaluated for narrowing and loculation. Another film is taken.
- Spillage of the contrast from the tubes into the peritoneal cavity is observed and evaluated. Another film is taken.
- The HSG catheter is then removed after its balloon has been deflated.
- All remaining instruments are removed.

Special Technique

- In some patients, the above-mentioned technique fails as a result of: (1) distorted cervical canal that prevents the flexible HSG catheter from passing into the uterine cavity or (2) a very narrow external os.
- In such cases a special HSG cannula with a plastic tip and a rubber cone, such as Kahn cannula (Novo Surgical Inc. Oak Brook, IL) can be used.
- The anterior lip of the cervix is grasped with the single-toothed tenaculum to enable manipulation and traction of the cervix.
- The syringe containing the contrast material is connected to the Kahn cannula.
- The cannula is then filled with the contrast material to avoid false positive results secondary to injecting air bubbles.
- The plastic tip of the cannula is then inserted into the cervical canal.
- The distal ends of the cannula and the tenaculum are then interlocked in a manner that allows maintenance of the tight seal when the contrast material is injected. The tenaculum and the cannula are removed at the end of the procedure.
- Hemostasis is ensured.

Complications

- Bleeding—at the site of tenaculum placement.
- Perforation—during placement of the flexible catheter (unlikely).
- Vasovagal reaction—during manipulation of the cervix or injection of contrast material.
- Contrast extravasation—during injection of the contrast material that may lead to oil embolism if oil-soluble contrast material is used.
- Infection—due to underlying subclinical infection or improper aseptic technique.
- Allergy reaction—to any component of the contrast material.

Interpretation

- Filled uterine cavity: evaluated for symmetry, shape, and presence of uterine septum or bicornuate uterus and unicornuate uterus.
- Filling defects, depending on the location:
  - Uterine cavity—may indicate uterine fibroid, polyp, or synechiae.
  - Cornu—may indicate occlusion versus spasm, or salpingitis isthmica nodosa.
  - Ampulla—may indicate intraluminal adhesions or tubal pregnancy.

- Fimbriated end—may indicate phimosis or hydrosalpinx.
- Loculation:
  - Tubal—may indicate partial occlusion or peritubal, periovarian or pelvic adhesions.
  - Peritoneal cavity—may indicate pelvic adhesions.

Accuracy

- HSG is considered a good screening test with high sensitivity.
- HSG has a low false positive rate.
- The accuracy of HSG depends on the technique and the experience of the operator.

Discussion with the Patient

The monitor will be activated and the results of the hysterosalpingogram will be shown to the patient and discussed with her and her family if they are present in the room. The patient will then be given an appointment in the office for further work-up.

BIBLIOGRAPHY

Acton, C.M., J.M. Devitt, and E.A. Ryan. 1988. "Hysterosalpingography in Infertility—an Experience of 3,631 Examinations." *Australian and New Zealand Journal of Obstetrics and Gynaecology* 28(2): 127–33.

Deboer, A.D., H.M. Vemer, W.N.P. Williamson, and F.V.M. Sanders. 1988. "All or Acquiesce Contrast Media for Hysterosalpingography: A Perspective, Randomized Clinical Study." *European Journal of Obstetrics and Gynecology and Reproductive Biology* 28(1): 65–8.

Furniss, H.D. 1921. "The Rubin Test Simplified." *Surgery, Gynecology & Obstetrics* 33: 567–8.

Lindequist, S., P. Justesen, C. Larsen, and F. Rasmussen. 1991. "Diagnostic Quality and Complications of Hysterosalpingography: Oil- Versus Water-Soluble Contrast Media: a Randomized Prospective Study." *Radiology* 179(1): 69–74.

Luttjeboer, F., T. Harada, E. Hughes, N. Johnson, R. Lilford, and B.W. Mol. 2007. "Tubal Flushing for Subfertility." *Cochrane Database of Systematic Reviews* CD003718.

Siegler, A.M. 1983. "Hysterosalpingography." *Fertility and Sterility* 40: 139.

Steinkeler, J.A., C.A. Woodfield, E. Lazarus, and N.N. Hillstrom. 2009. "Female Infertility, A Systematic Approach to Radiologic Imaging and Diagnosis." *Radiographics* 29: 1353–70.

51

Intrauterine Insemination: Clinical Perspectives

Willem Ombelet

Rationale for Intrauterine Insemination (IUI)

- To increase the number of motile spermatozoa at the site of fertilization.
- Non-invasive technique of assisted reproduction.
- IUI with ovarian stimulation is cost-effective as a first-line therapy when compared to IVF in unexplained subfertility and moderate male subfertility cases.

Indications

- Cervical factor subfertility
- Retrograde ejaculation
- Anatomical factors
- Unexplained subfertility
- Moderate male factor subfertility

Contraindications

- Bilateral tubal block
- Severe male sub(in)fertility

Pre-Treatment Assessment

- Endocrine investigation
- Transvaginal 2D ultrasound (ovarian reserve assessment, ovarian cysts, congenital uterine malformations)
- Hysterosalpingography/ultrasonography
- Diagnostic hysteroscopy in selected cases
- Laparoscopy in selected cases (unexplained long-standing infertility, suspicion of endometriosis/ovarian cysts/adhesions)
- Semen analysis in native sample
- Semen analysis after sperm washing

Evidence-Based Recommendations

- IUI for cervical factor: natural cycle IUI is recommended
- Unexplained infertility or mild endometriosis: no IUI (conservative management) or IUI with ovarian stimulation
- Moderate male subfertility: IUI success increases if:
  - Sperm morphology >4%
  - Inseminating motile count (IMC) >1 million
  - Total motile sperm count native sample >5 million
  - Total motility in native sample >30%
- IUI success rate significantly increases with the use of hMG/rec FSH—save multiple pregnancy rates
- IUI success rate significantly increases if endometrial thickness ≥6.3 mm and/or triple layer image at the moment of HCG triggering
- Optimal time-interval between HCG-trigger and IUI: 12–36 hours
- Double IUI (2 IUIs per cycle): can be indicated in male subfertility cases
- Immobilization after IUI: 10–15 minutes

Sperm Preparation for IUI: Required Equipment

- Laminar flow hood, class II
- Incubator with appropriate % CO_2
- Centrifuge with swing-out rotor
- Phase-contrast microscope
- Heating stage as working stage under the microscope
- Heating plate
- Makler counting chamber
- Sterile pipettes for handling sperm samples: 1 mL, 5 mL, 10 mL
- Conical 15 mL tubes
- Waste recipient
- 5 mL tubes

- Gloves: either
  - PureSperm Wash
    - PureSperm 80 gradient
    - PureSperm 40 gradient or
  - Nidacon Sperm Wash
    - P80 gradient Nidacon
    - P40 gradient Nidacon
    - Proinsert Nidacon

Sperm Preparation for IUI: Method 1 (PureSperm Wash)

- Put PureSperm Wash and gradients 80 and 40 into the laminar flow hood at room temperature at least 30 minutes before starting.
- Make the PureSperm gradient by pipetting 2 mL of gradient 80 into a 15 mL conical tube. Add 2 mL of gradient 40 very gently on top of gradient 80 by pipetting it very slowly at the side of the tube without mixing the two layers. Make as many tubes as necessary (max 1.5 mL sperm sample per gradient tube).
- Prepare 2×5 mL of PureSperm Wash per patient in a 15 mL tube.
- Identify patient/sperm sample and label appropriately all tubes where necessary.
- Wait for total sperm liquidation before starting the procedure (±30 minutes).
- Wear gloves.
- All manipulations with the sperm sample are performed within the laminar flow hood.
- Measure the volume of the sperm sample into a pipette and pipette very gently a 1 mL–1.5 mL sample on top of the PureSperm gradients.
- Save 100 µL of the sample and put it in a 5 mL tube for counting sperm motility and concentration.
- Centrifuge the gradients for 20 minutes at 300 g.
- Put the tubes into the laminar flow hood again and pipette the upper gradient layers by moving the point of the pipette in a circle. Collect this debris into a waste collection recipient. Keep 0.3 mL of the sperm pellet of each tube and pipette this into the 5 mL PureSperm Wash solution.
- Centrifuge again for 10 minutes at 500 g.
- Remove the upper layer again and re-suspend the sperm pellet into the second tube of 5 mL PureSperm Wash solution.
- Centrifuge again for 10 minutes at 500 g.
- Again remove the upper layer and re-suspend the sperm pellet in 0.7 mL of PureSperm Wash Solution. Take a small drop out of this sample for counting sperm motility and concentration after capacitation.
- Equilibrate at least 15 minutes before performing the IUI.

Sperm Preparation for IUI: Method 2 (Using ProInsert)

- Put Sperm Wash and gradients P80 and P40 into the laminar flow hood at room temperature at least 30 minutes before starting.
- Take the number of centrifuge tubes with ProInsert needed according to the volume to be capacitated (max 1.5 mL sperm sample per gradient tube).
- Use a serological pipette to add 2 mL of PureSperm 80 to the outer channel. The gradient will run down into the ProInsert Chamber, out through a hole at the bottom of the chamber, and down the wall of the centrifuge tube to form a layer at the bottom of the centrifuge tube.
- Repeat the step above using a new pipette and P40 according to manufacturer's specifications, again to the outer channel.
- Make as many tubes as necessary.
- Prepare 2×5 mL of PureSperm Wash per patient in a 15 mL tube.
- Identify patient/sperm sample and label appropriately all tubes where necessary.
- Wait for total sperm liquidation before starting the procedure (±30 minutes).
- Wear gloves.
- All manipulations with the sperm sample are performed within the laminar flow hood.
- Measure the volume of the sperm sample into a pipette and pipette very gently a 1 mL–1.5 mL sample on top of the PureSperm gradients into the outer channel, taking care not to touch the edges of the central channel with the semen.
- Save 100 µL of the sample and put it in a 5 mL tube for counting sperm motility and concentration.
- Centrifuge the gradients for 20 minutes at 300 g.
- Put the tubes into the laminar flow hood again.
- Attach the sperm-retrieval pipette from the ProInsert kit to a 1 mL syringe.
- Pass the pipette slowly into the ProInsert via the central channel, down to the sperm pellet, taking care not to disrupt the pellet. Aspirate 200 µL of the sperm pellet and retract the pipette until the tip of the pipette is safely above the liquid surface; aspirate some air and retract the pipette from the central channel. Transfer the pellet into the 5 mL PureSperm Wash solution.
- Centrifuge again for 10 minutes at 500 g.
- Remove the upper layer again and re-suspend the sperm pellet in 5 mL of PureSperm Wash solution.
- Centrifuge again for 10 minutes at 500 g.
- Again remove the upper layer and re-suspend the sperm pellet in 0.7 mL of PureSperm Wash solution. Take a small drop out of this sample for

counting sperm motility and concentration after sperm preparation.

• Equilibrate at least 15 minutes before performing the IUI.

BIBLIOGRAPHY

Bensdorp A.J., R.I. Tjon-Kon-Fat, P.M. Bossuyt, C.A. Koks, G.J. Oosterhuis, A. Hoek, et al. 2015. "Prevention Of Multiple Pregnancies in Couples with Unexplained or Mild Male Subfertility: Randomised Controlled Trial of in Vitro Fertilisation with Single Embryo Transfer or in Vitro Fertilisation in Modified Natural Cycle Compared with Intrauterine Insemination with Controlled Ovarian Hyperstimulation." *BMJ* Jan 9: 350: g7771. doi: 10.1136/bmj.g7771.

Cohlen, B. and Ombelet W. (eds). 2014. *Intra-Uterine Insemination: Evidence-Based Guidelines for Daily Practice*. Boca Raton, FL: CRC Press.

Ombelet W., H. Vandeput, G. Van de Putte, A. Cox, M. Janssen, P. Jacobs, et al. 1997. "Intrauterine Insemination After Ovarian Stimulation with Clomiphene Citrate: Predictive Potential of Inseminating Motile Count and Sperm Morphology?" *Human Reproduction* 12: 1458–63.

Ombelet W., N. Dhont, A. Thijssen, E. Bosmans, and T. Kruger. 2014. "Semen Quality and Prediction of IUI Success in Male Subfertility: A Systematic Review." *Reproductive Biomedicine Online* 28: 300–9.

52

GnRH Agonist to Trigger Final Follicular Maturation in IVF

Nayana Talukdar and Robert F. Casper

Introduction

Ovarian hyperstimulation syndrome (OHSS) is one of the major concerns of controlled ovarian stimulation (COS) in an IVF cycle. High-risk patients include those with polycystic ovarian syndrome (PCOS), multi-follicular ovarian morphology on ultrasound, or those who have actually developed OHSS in previous stimulated cycles.[1] Since the standard human chorionic gonadotrophin (hCG) trigger produces a prolonged luteotrophic effect that may promote OHSS, withholding the ovulatory dose of hCG is the best option to avoid OHSS, but results in cycle cancellation associated with significant social, emotional and economic factors. In addition, some of these cycles might not have progressed to OHSS if triggered with hCG. Hence, as an alternative to the conventional hCG trigger, the concept of using a bolus dose of GnRH agonist (GnRHa) for triggering ovulation in patients "at risk" has become the standard of care for high responders in GnRH antagonist cycles.[1]

GnRHa

- GnRHa has been used to induce final oocyte maturation and trigger ovulation since the early 1990s, both in IVF and non-IVF cycles in which COS is used.[2,3]
- GnRHa acts upon the anterior pituitary gland to release LH and FSH, similar to the spontaneous mid-cycle gonadotropin surge.
- The short half-life of LH (60 minutes compared to 24 hours for hCG) along with pituitary desensitization leads to luteolysis, hence eliminating or dramatically reducing the risk of OHSS.
- However, GnRHa triggering can only be used in cycles where GnRH antagonist is used to suppress the gonadotropin surge.
- Because of the higher affinity of GnRH receptors to GnRH agonists than GnRH antagonists, the pituitary remains responsive to GnRHa in IVF cycles in which GnRH antagonist protocols are used.

Doses of GnRH Agonist

The published bolus doses of different GnRHa, when used as a trigger are: leuprolide acetate (Lupron) 0.5 to 4 mg subcutaneously, triptorelin (Decapeptyl) 0.2 mg subcutaneously and buserelin (Suprefact) 0.5 mg subcutaneously.

Prevention of OHSS Studies

- In high-risk patients stimulated for IVF with an antagonist protocol, none of the patients triggered with GnRHa developed OHSS, compared to 31% in the hCG-triggered group.[1]
- In another study, the use of a GnRHa trigger was associated with a lower incidence of moderate/severe OHSS in the donors (0% versus 1.26% with an hCG trigger), while the recipient implantation and pregnancy rates per embryo transfer were comparable with either trigger.[4]

Luteal Phase Deficiency and Management

- Although the efficacy of the GnRHa trigger as a novel way to prevent OHSS is clear, poor implantation and pregnancy rates discouraged its use in IVF cycles.
- Maintaining a serum estrogen level of more than 200 pg/mL (725 pmol/L) and a progesterone level of more than 20 ng/mL (65 nmol/L) with "enhanced" or "aggressive" luteal support gives comparable implantation rates (36% vs. 31%) and clinical pregnancy rates (56.7% vs. 51.7%) with fresh embryo transfer in GnRHa versus hCG triggered cycles, respectively.[1]
- An example of the enhanced luteal support is progesterone (100 mg IM daily with vaginal progesterone 200 mg) or estrogen and progesterone (micronised progesterone gel 90 mg twice daily, plus 2 mg oral estradiol thrice daily).

- The requirement for a high replacement doses of estradiol and progesterone led to various combination protocols for support of the luteal phase in GnRHa triggered cycles, either by high-dose steroid supplementation or by minimal stimulation of the corpus luteum.

    - In one such protocol, a "dual trigger" with GnRHa together with low-dose hCG (≤15 IU/lb body weight or up to 1500 IU) 36 hours prior to oocyte retrieval, along with aggressive estrogen and progesterone supplementation (see below), has been found to improve pregnancy rates compared to using the GnRHa trigger alone.

    - The concept is to simulate the actions of LH in the early luteal phase to support implantation and luteal ovarian steroidogenesis.[5]

    - In "low-risk patients" (less than 12 follicles >12 mm), 1500 IU HCG administered on the day of retrieval and again 4 days later, without any additional luteal support, was found to result in good pregnancy rates.[6]

Segmentation of IVF Cycles

- By far the most favored strategy to deal with both high-risk OHSS and luteal phase insufficiency is the "freeze-all" strategy, also termed "segmentation" of the IVF cycle.[7]

- In this strategy, COS with GnRHa trigger is followed by vitrification of embryos/oocytes in one cycle, and frozen embryo transfer in subsequent thaw cycles.

- This strategy is feasible provided there is access to an optimal cryopreservation program.

- Such an approach protects the embryo and the endometrium from the detrimental effects of supraphysiological levels of hormones reached during the ovarian stimulation process.

REFERENCES

1. L. Engmann, A. DiLuigi, D. Schmidt, J. Nulsen, D. Maier, and C. Benadiva, "The Use of Gonadotropin-Releasing Hormone (GnRH) Agonist to Induce Oocyte Maturation After Cotreatment with Gnrh Antagonist in High-Risk Patients Undergoing in Vitro Fertilization Prevents the Risk of Ovarian Hyperstimulation Syndrome: A Prospective Randomized Controlled Study," *Fertility and Sterility* 89 (2008): 84–91.

2. Y. Gonen, H. Balakier, W. Powell, and R.F. Casper, "Use of Gonadotropin-Releasing Hormone Agonist to Trigger Follicular Maturation for in Vitro Fertilization," *J Clinical Endocrinology & Metabolism* 71 (1990): 918–22.

3. J. Itskovitz, R. Boldes, J. Levron, Y. Erlik, L. Kahana, J.M. Brandes, "Induction of Preovulatory Luteinizing Hormone Surge and Prevention of Ovarian Hyperstimulation Syndrome by Gonadotropin-Releasing Hormone Agonist," *Fertility and Sterility* 56 (1991): 213–20.

4. D. Bodri, J.J. Guillen, A. Galindo, D. Mataro, A. Pujol, O. Coll, "Triggering with Human Chorionic Gonadotrophin or a Gonadotrophin-Releasing Hormone Agonist in Gonadotrophin-Releasing Hormone Antagonist-Treated Oocyte Donor Cycles: Findings of a Large Retrospective Cohort Study," *Fertility and Sterility* 91 (2009): 365–71.

5. B.S. Shapiro, S.T. Daneshmand, F.C. Garner, M. Aguirre, and C. Hudson, "Comparison of 'Triggers' Using Leuprolide Acetate Alone or in Combination with Low-Dose Human Chorionic Gonadotropin," *Fertility and Sterility* 95 (2011): 2715–17.

6. S. Kol, P. Humaidan, J. Itskovitz-Eldor, "GnRH agonist ovulation trigger and hCG-based, Progesterone-Free Luteal Support: A Proof of Concept Study," *Human Reproduction* 26 (2011): 2874–7.

7. P. Devroey, N.P. Polyzos, and C. Blockeel, "An OHSS-Free Clinic by Segmentation of IVF Treatment," *Human Reproduction* 26 (2011): 2593–7.

53

GnRH Agonist Protocols

Justin Tan, Rabea Youcef Khoudja, Michael Dooley, Michael H. Dahan, and Seang Lin Tan

Mechanism of Action of GnRH Agonists

- GnRH agonists stimulate the pituitary gland to produce a rise in follicle-stimulating hormone (FSH) and LH, which then peaks after several hours and declines with continued administration of the GnRH agonists, so usually within a few days (3–4 days) patients will have a refractory response to continued FSH/LH stimulation.
- There are a number of GnRH agonists protocols:
  - Long protocol: This protocol remains the most commonly used protocol in the world today.
    - There are basically two variations: (1) commencement of the GnRH agonist in the early follicular phase or (2) commencement in the mid-luteal phase of the preceding cycle.
    - In both cases, scheduling can be done more easily by the addition of oral contraceptive pills for a few weeks before the addition of the GnRH agonists.[1]
    - The advantage of the mid-luteal phase start is that generally the incidence of cyst formation after pituitary suppression is less than with early follicular phase start.
    - When suppression is confirmed, gonadotropins are commenced and the buserelin dose is lowered to 200 mcg/day (buserelin continues at this dose until and including the day of hCG); if leuprolide is taken, the dose is reduced to 200 mcg/day.
    - The starting dose of gonadotropins will depend on patient's age, ovarian function or previous response to gonadotropins. For a first cycle, doses should conform to the following:
      - 100–150 IU HMG/FSH <30 years.
      - 150–225 IU HMG/FSH 30–38 years.
      - 225–300 IU HMG/FSH 39–40 years.
      - 300–450 IU HMG/FSH >40 years.
      - If a patient has PCOS, use a daily dose that is 75 IU less than would be normally ordered. If FSH is >10, use a higher dose than would be normally ordered.
      - **Note:** The maximum dose of FSH is 600 IU/day. Use the effective dose of the HMG/FSH in a previous cycle as the starting dose in subsequent cycles. If estradiol in a previous cycle was low in relation to number of follicles, give LH (ideally, in a ratio of 3:1).
      - Several ultrasound scans are performed and estradiol measurements are individualized.
      - When the biggest follicles reach an average mean diameter of 17–18 mm or more, with 3 follicles of 18 mm, hCG is administered and egg collection is scheduled 34–38 hours later.
      - A major advantage of the long protocol is flexible timing of the hCG within a 2–3 day window.[2]
  - Short protocol: Buserelin was administered from day 2 and HMG or FSH from day 3 of the menstrual cycle, and both continued until the day of hCG administration.
  - Ultrashort protocol: Buserelin was administered on days 2, 3, and 4, and HMG or FSH was given from day 3 of the cycle until the day of hCG administration.[3]
  - Ultra-long protocol: This protocol uses prolonged pituitary suppression for a few months (typically 3 cycles of depot-lupron or decapeptyl) before stimulation begins. It has been shown to be particularly useful for patients with stage 3 or 4 endometriosis.[4,5]

Table 53.1 shows the long protocol vs. antagonist cycles in women <35, FSH <10, first IVF, good responders (data from Grow et al.).[6]

Table 53.2 shows the long protocol vs. antagonist cycles in women <35, FSH <10 in first IVF for good responders: the

TABLE 53.1

Characteristics	Stimulation Protocol	
	Agonist + FSH (n = 16,001)	Antagonist + FSH (n = 7112)
Age (mean ± SD)	30.4 ± 2.7	30.5 ± 2.8
Implantation rate (%)	8331 (57.6)	3403 (54.1), (p <0.05)
Live births for all cycles (%)	52.6	49.2, (p <0.05)
eSET cycles (%)	1489 (10.85)	767 (12.87), (p <0.05)
Live birth in eSET cycles (%)	53.93	46.15, (p <0.05)
Moderate OHSS (%)	342 (2.1)	120 (1.7), (p <0.05)
Severe OHSS (%)	118 (0.7)	42 (0.6)

TABLE 53.2

	Odds Ratio (Confidence Interval)	Adjusted Odds Ratio (Confidence Interval)
All good prognosis completed cycles		
Implantation	1.15 (1.04 to 1.27)	1.14 (1.03 to 1.26)
Live birth	1.14 (1.04 to 1.26)	1.13 (1.03 to 1.25)
All cycles with elective SET		
Implantation	1.41 (1.13 to 1.76)	1.36 (1.08 to 1.73)
Live birth	1.37 (1.11 to 1.68)	1.33 (1.07 to 1.66)

long protocol has better results than antagonist (data from Grow et al.).[6]

GnRH Agonist Protocol vs. GnRH Antagonist Protocol

Because of the need for prolonged treatment cycles and more complex treatments for patients, there has been a move to a more patient-friendly GnRH antagonist protocol, which has similar live birth rates.

The Use of GnRH Agonists for Down-Regulation for Frozen Embryo Transfer Cycles

It has been shown that unless a cyst forms or the growth of follicles is from the use of Estrace, GnRH agonist down-regulation is not necessary for HRT-FERC cycles.[5]

REFERENCES

1. M.M. Biljan, N.G. Mahutte, N. Dean, R. Hemmings, F. Bissonnette, and S.L. Tan, "Effects of Pre-Treatment with an Oral Contraceptive on the Time Required to Achieve Pituitary Suppression with Gonadotropin-Releasing Hormone Analogues and Subsequent Implantation and Pregnancy Rates," *Fertility and Sterility* 70 (1998): 1063–9.

2. S.L. Tan, O. Royston, S. Campbell, H.S. Jacobs, J. Betts, B.A. Mason, R.G. Edwards. "Cumulative Conception and Livebirth Rates After In-Vitro Fertilization," *Lancet*, 339 (1992): 1390–4.

3. S.L. Tan, N. Maconochie, P. Doyle, S. Campbell, A. Balen, J. Bekir, P. Brinsden, R.G. Edwards, and H.S. Jacobs, "Cumulative Conception and Live-Birth Rates After In Vitro Fertilization With and Without the Use of Long, Short, and Ultrashort Regimens of the Gonadotropin-Releasing Hormone Agonist Buserelin," *American Journal of Obstetrics and Gynecology* 171 (1994): 513–20.

4. J. Ren, A. Sha, D. Han, P. Li, J. Geng, and C. Ma, "Does Prolonged Pituitary Down-Regulation with Gonadotropin-Releasing Hormone Agonist Improve the Live-Birth Rate in in Vitro Fertilization Treatment?" *Fertility and Sterility* 102(1) (2014): 75–81.

5. A. van de Vijver, N.P. Polyzos, L. Van Landuyt, M. De Vos, M. Camus, D. Stoop, H. Tournaye, and C. Blockeel, "Cryopreserved Embryo Transfer in an Artificial Cycle: Is GnRH Agonist Down-Regulation Necessary?" *Reproductive Biomedicine Online* 29(5) (2014): 588–94.

6. D. Grow, J.F. Kawwass, A.D. Kulkarni, T. Durant, D.J. Jamieson, and M. Macaluso, "GnRH Agonist and GnRH Antagonist Protocols: Comparison of Outcomes Among Good-Prognosis Patients Using National Surveillance Data," *Reproductive BioMedicine* 29 (2014): 299–304.

54

GnRH Agonists before IVF for Advanced Endometriosis

Hassan N. Sallam and Nooman H. Sallam

Endometriosis and IVF

Women with endometriosis who are treated with in vitro fertilization (IVF) or intracytoplasmic sperm injection (ICSI) have a lower clinical pregnancy rate compared to women with tubal factor infertility.[1] Additionally, patients with advanced endometriosis (ASRM stages III and IV) have significantly lower clinical pregnancy rates compared to those with minimal and mild endometriosis (stages I and II). Whether this association is due to a defect in the oocytes or in the endometrium or in both has been a subject of debate.[2,3]

Surgery before IVF in Advanced Endometriosis

The role of surgery before IVF in advanced endometriosis is still controversial.[4,5,6] The following indications for endometrioma resection before IVF have been proposed: (1) no prior surgical confirmation of endometriosis, (2) severe pelvic pain attributable to mass, (3) rapid growth, (4) suspicious sonographic features, (5) compromised access to remaining follicles, and (6) concern for rupture in pregnancy due to size.[6]

Medical Approaches to Treat Advanced Endometriosis before IVF

Medical approaches prior to IVF in patients with advanced endometriosis are an alternative option and many have been suggested. They include corticosteroids,[7] Danazol,[8] oral contraceptives,[9] and GnRH agonists.[10]

GnRH Agonists before IVF

In our meta-analysis of randomized studies using long-term GnRH agonists prior to IVF, we have found that this approach is associated with a 4-fold increase in the clinical pregnancy rate.[10] We have also found that the live birth rate was increased 9-fold, although this finding was based on only one of the studies.[10]

Protocol

- The first injection of the long-term GnRH agonist should be given during the early follicular phase and repeated every 28 days.
- One of the following preparations can be used for this purpose:
  - A depot preparation of the GnRH agonist leuprotide acetate 3.75 mg given by the IM route.
  - A depot preparation of the GnRH agonist goserelin, 3.6 mg, given by the SC route.
  - A depot preparation of the GnRH agonist D-tryptorelin microcapsule 3.2 mg by the IM route.
- Controlled ovarian hyperstimulation should be initiated 30 to 45 days after the third injection by the daily administration of the short-acting GnRH agonist.
  - For example, leuprolide acetate 0.5 to 1.0 mg/day can be started by SC injection for 7 to 10 days.
  - Once gonadotropin suppression is confirmed, the dose should be reduced to 0.25 to 0.5 mg/d SC and exogenous gonadotropin stimulation should be started and IVF or ICSI conducted in the usual fashion.
- Alternatively, GnRH antagonist protocol may be initiated 30 days after the last GnRH depot injection with the IM administration of the gonadotropins and the IVF or ICSI conducted in the usual fashion.

Conclusions

In patients with advanced endometriosis, long-term administration of GnRH agonists before IVF is associated with a significant increase in clinical pregnancy. Based on currently available evidence, women with endometriosis treated with IVF or ICSI should receive GnRH agonist therapy for a minimum of three months prior to the procedure as this will increase the odds of clinical pregnancy 4-fold, bearing in mind that data regarding adverse effects of this therapy on the mother or fetus are not available at present.

REFERENCES

1. K. Barnhart, R. Dunsmoor-Su, and C. Coutifaris, "Effect of Endometriosis on in Vitro Fertilization," *Fertility and Sterility* 77 (2002): 1148–55.

2. A. Pellicer, J. Navarro, E. Bosch, N. Garrido, J.A. García-Velasco, J. Remohi, et al., "Endometrial Quality in Infertile Women with Endometriosis." *Annals of the New York Academy of Science* 943 (2001): 122–30.

3. A.M. Mohamed, S. Chouliaras, C.J. Jones, and L.G. Nardo, "Live Birth Rate in Fresh and Frozen Embryo Transfer Cycles in Women with Endometriosis" *European Journal of Obstetrics & Gynecology and Reproductive Biology* 156 (2011): 177–80.

4. P.H. Bianchi, R.M. Pereira, A. Zanatta, J.R. Alegretti, E.L. Motta, and P.C. Serafini, "Extensive Excision of Deep Infiltrative Endometriosis Before in Vitro Fertilization Significantly Improves Pregnancy Rates." *Journal of Minimally Invasive Gynecology* 16 (2009): 174–80.

5. I. Tsoumpou, M. Kyrgiou, T.A. Gelbaya, and L.G. Nardo, "The Effect of Surgical Treatment for Endometrioma on in Vitro Fertilization Outcomes: A Systematic Review and Meta-Analysis." *Fertility and Sterility* 92 (2009): 75–87.

6. J.A. García-Velasco and E. Somigliana. "Management of Endometriomas in Women Requiring IVF: To Touch or Not to Touch." *Human Reproduction* 24(3) (2009): 496–501.

7. C.H. Kim, H.D. Chae, B.M. Kang, Y.S. Chang, and J.E. Mok, "The Immunotherapy During in Vitro Fertilization and Embryo Transfer Cycles in Infertile Patients with Endometriosis." *Journal of Obstetric and Gynaecologic Research* 23 (1997): 463–70.

8. C. Tei, T. Miyazaki, N. Kuji, M. Tanaka, K. Sueoka, and Y. Yoshimura. "Effect of Danazol on the Pregnancy Rate in Patients with Unsuccessful in Vitro Fertilization-Embryo Transfer." *Journal of Reproductive Medicine* 43(6) (1998): 541–6.

9. D. de Ziegler, V. Gayet, F.X. Aubriot, P. Fauque, I. Streuli, J.P. Wolf, J. de Mouzon, and C. Chapron. "Use of Oral Contraceptives in Women with Endometriosis Before Assisted Reproduction Treatment Improves Outcomes." *Fertility and Sterility* 94(7) (2010): 2796–9.

10. H.N. Sallam, J.A. Garcia-Velasco, S. Dias, A. Arici, and A.M. Abou-Setta, "Long-Term Pituitary Down-Regulation Before in Vitro Fertilization (IVF) for Women with Endometriosis." *Cochrane Database of Systematic Reviews* 1 (2006): CD004635.

55

Microdose GnRH Agonist Flare Protocol

Magued Adel Mikhail, Wael Salem, and Botros Rizk

Introduction

Patients with poor ovarian reserve represent between 9%–24% of the population in IVF centers. Poor responders present multiple challenges in achieving optimal oocyte quality and quantity, while minimizing cycle cancellation rates in order to achieve adequate pregnancy rates. Overall, poor responders experience decreased oocyte yields, fertilization rates, pregnancy and live birth rates.

The approach to improve outcomes among poor responders has involved increasing gonadotropin dose, reducing GnRH agonist dose, estrogen priming, and a long flare protocol utilizing both GnRH agonist and gonadotropins in parallel.

The microdose flare protocol was first described in 1994 as an alternative to the long flare protocol as it demonstrated improved oocyte yield, decreased cycle cancellation, decreased premature LH surges, and improved pregnancy rates.

This chapter highlights the benefits of a microdose flare (MDF) with specific attention to appropriate patient selection and protocol technique.

Microdose Flare

- The initial studies investigating the MDF protocol demonstrated a higher oocyte yield and ongoing pregnancy rate in paired controlled trials comparing the patients' previous cycles to cycles with MDF.
- The benefits of a MDF are believed to be largely attributable to an enhanced endogenous release of FSH during the early follicular phase.
- One of the most important determinants of successful utilization of MDF is appropriate selection of patients.
- Among women with diminished ovarian reserve, a MDF is likely most beneficial for women with low ovarian volume, decreased antral follicle counts and a low anti-Mullerian hormone level.

Protocol

- Generally, the patient is pretreated with a combined oral contraceptive pill to reduce the risk of corpus luteum rescue and the subsequent harmful effects of a rise in progesterone and androgens.
- A twice daily injection of leuprolide acetate 20 mcg daily is started on cycle day 3.
- Gonadotropins are then started on cycle day 5.
- Growth hormone is initiated on cycle day 6, because evidence from multiple trials indicates that the addition of GH is associated with an increased pregnancy rate.

Gonadotropin Stimulation

- Stratification of the patient's risk factors for a poor response should take into account her age and ovarian reserve markers.
- Pending this clinical decision making, the appropriate dose is generally between 300 and 450 IU of rFSH.
- It is important to note that there is controversy regarding the use of doses greater than 300 IU of rFSH, as a previous prospective randomized study demonstrated no improvement in outcomes with doses greater than 300 IU.

Trigger

- When follicles reach 18 mm in average diameter, an HCG trigger may be administered for final maturation of the oocytes.

Luteal Phase Support

- The use of luteal phase support with vaginal or intramuscular progesterone has been widely described in the literature as imperative to a stimulated IVF cycle.

- For natural micronized progesterone, doses of 300–600 mg split into two or three administrations daily may be administered vaginally.
- For intramuscular progesterone, a dose of 25–100 mg/day may be utilized.
- Luteal phase support is generally started no earlier than the day of oocyte retrieval and no later than day 5 following administration of HCG trigger.

Conclusion

The management of poor responders remains controversial and an ideal protocol has not yet been demonstrated to work for poor responders as a group.

- An adequate protocol should ideally lead to an optimal number of oocytes and good-quality embryos while minimizing cycle cancellation rates in order to maximize pregnancy and live birth rates.
- The microdose GnRH agonist flare-up protocol was developed to exploit the release of endogenous gonadotropin through administration of a low-dose GnRH agonist.
- This protocol has been demonstrated to increase oocyte yield while minimizing premature LH surge and cycle cancellation effectively leading to higher pregnancy rates among poor responders.
- For the appropriately selected patient, microdose GnRH agonist protocol offers multiple benefits to an ovarian stimulation protocol while minimizing unwanted outcomes.

BIBLIOGRAPHY

Aboulghar, M. "Role of GnRH Antagonist in Assisted Reproduction." In *Ovarian Stimulation*, edited by M. Abulghar and B. Risk, 49–60. Cambridge: Cambridge University Press, 2011.

Berkkanoglu, M., and K. Ozgur. 2010. "What Is the Optimum Maximal Gonadotropin Dosage Used in Microdose Flare-Up Cycles in Poor Responders?" *Fertility and Sterility* 94(2): 662–5. doi: 10.1016/j.fertnstert.2009.03.027. Epub 2009 Apr 14.

Cheong, Y., N. Brook, and N. Macklon. "New Concepts in Ovarian Stimulation." In *Human-assisted Reproductive Technology*, edited by D.K. Gardner, B.R.M.B. Risk, and T. Falcon, 55–72. Cambridge: Cambridge University Press, 2011.

Keay, S.D., N.H. Liversedge, R.S. Mathur, and J.M. Jenkins. 1997. "Assisted Conception Following Poor Ovarian Response to Gonadotrophin Stimulation." *British Journal of Obstetrics and Gynaecology* 104: 521–7.

Kolibianakis, E.M., and G. Griesienger. "GnRH Antagonist in ART." In *Human-assisted Reproductive Technology*, edited by D.K. Gardner, B.R.M.B. Risk, and T. Falcon, 73–79. Cambridge: Cambridge University Press, 2011.

Schoolcraft, W., T. Sclenker, M. Gee, J. Stevens, and L. Wagley. 1997. "Improved Controlled Ovarian Hyperstimulation in Poor Responder in Vitro Fertilization Patients with a Microdose Follicle-Stimulating Hormone Flare, Growth Hormone Protocol." *Fertility and Sterility* 67: 93–7.

Scott, R., and D. Navot. 1994. "Enhancement of Ovarian Responsiveness with Microdoses of Gonadotropin-Releasing Hormone Agonists During Ovulation Induction for in Vitro Fertilization." *Fertility and Sterility* 61: 880–5.

Surrey, E.S., J. Bower, D.M. Hill, J. Ramsey, and M.W. Surrey. 1998. "Clinical and Endocrine Effects of a Microdose GnRH Agonist Flare Regimen Administered to Poor Responders Who Are Undergoing in Vitro Fertilization." *Fertility and Sterility* 69(3): 419–24.

56

Gonadotropin-Releasing Hormone Antagonist Cycle for In Vitro Fertilization

Michael H. Dahan, Justin Tan, Baris Ata, Rabea Youcef Khoudja, and Seang Lin Tan

Introduction

Application of the GnRH antagonist (GnRH-AT) IVF cycle has been used in two populations:

- Those at risk of developing OHSS (high responders)
- Poor responders to ovarian stimulation

Two regimens of GnRH-AT are available:

- A daily dose (250 mcg of Ganeralix or Cetrorelix)
- A dose with three days' effect (3 mg Cetrorelix)

GnRH-AT IVF Cycle

- Stimulation is initiated with gonadotropins on cycle day 2–3.
- High responders: Starting dose 100–225 IU daily based on age, body weight, AFC, AMH, and previous response.
- Poor responders: Starting dose 300–600 IU daily based on clinic maximum dose guidelines.
- If patient weighs more than 170 lbs (77.1 kg), add an additional 75 IU of gonadotropin.
- Addition of 75 IU-225 IU daily of LH activity should be considered.
- Traditionally, FSH to LH activity should be 2:1 or 3:1.[1]

The GnRH-AT Can Be Initiated Per Two Protocols

- Variable start: when lead follicle is 12–14 mm (ideally 3–4 days of antagonist are given as maximum).
- Fixed start: GnRH-AT initiated 4–6 days after gonadotropins started.

Ultrasound Monitoring (Transvaginal)

- On cycle day (CD) two or three, verify no new ovarian cysts present larger than 1.5 cm or serum estradiol >100 pmol/L. If present, cancel cycle and wait until next.
- Repeat ultrasound by day 5 for variable-start cycles or by day 7 for fixed cycles.
- Ultrasound is performed every 1–3 days based on lead follicle size.
- Serum estradiol levels often drop when GnRH-AT is initiated, but this is not associated with negative outcomes. However, some authors will increase the dose of gonadotropins by 75 IU.

Trigger for Collection

- When two 17 mm follicles present; and
- When at least 50% of follicles are 10–20 mm (as measured by mean diameter). If fresh ET is contemplated, then hCG trigger should not be delayed after above criteria achieved.[2]

Trigger for Collection 34–38 Hours before Egg Retrieval

- Trigger can be accomplished with hCG 5000 to 10,000 IU or recombinant hCG 250 μg dose.

Benefits of GnRH-AT Cycles over Other Cycles for High Responders

- A dose of GnRH agonist can be used instead of hCG to trigger ovulation.
  - Traditionally 500 μg to 1000 μg Buserelin or Luprolide acetate 1 mg is given.

- However, unless all embryos are being frozen for FERC, intensive luteal support or a small dose of hCG 1500 IU has to be given to support the luteal phase.[3]
- If more than 15 oocytes are collected, all embryos should be frozen and transferred in a subsequent frozen cycle.[4]
- If risk of OHSS is not excessive, and fewer than 15 oocytes were collected, consider adding 1500 IU of hCG after oocyte collection or adding intensive luteal support and performing a fresh embryo transfer.[5]
- Alternative luteal support strategies to permit fresh transfer after GnRH agonist trigger:
  - 100 mg progesterone in oil daily as a muscular injection and estradiol valerate 2 mg three times daily starting the night of collection.[6]
  - hCG 500 IU subcutaneous injection every three days evening after oocyte retrieval.

Fresh Embryo Transfer in GnRH-AT Cycles

- Regardless of trigger approach: progesterone luteal support starting on night of oocyte retrieval

Oocyte Donor

- Use of GnRH-AT with GnRH agonist trigger can be used to minimize risk of OHSS for the donor. To maximize number of oocytes, trigger can be done when largest follicle is 20 mm.
- Pre-treatment with less than 30 days of oral contraceptive pills can be used to synchronize the cycle with the oocyte recipient.
- Use of oral contraceptive pretreatment decreases stimulation, therefore an increase in gonadotropin stimulating dose by 75 IU may be considered.

Poor Responders

- Pretreatment with luteal phase estrogen before initiation of the GnRH-AT cycle may be attempted.
- Start estrogen (Estrace 4–6 mg daily or estradiol patches changed every other day) 5–7 days after spontaneous LH surge. Discontinue on CD 2 of spontaneous menses.
- Transvaginal ultrasound to measure follicles CD 3 and initiate gonadotropin stimulation.

Unique Possibilities for Poor Responders with the GnRH-AT Cycle

- An aromatase inhibitor or clomiphene citrate can be started on CD 2 for 5 days.
  - Gonadotropin can then be added on CD 4.
- Antagonist initiated CD 8, assuming folliculogenesis of 12–14 mm has occurred.[6,7]

REFERENCES

1. L. Engmann, A. Shaker, E. White, J.S. Bekir, H.S. Jacobs, S.L. Tan. "A Prospective Randomized Study to Assess the Clinical Efficacy of Gonadotrophins Administered Subcutaneously and Intramuscularly," *Human Reproduction*, 13 (1998): 836–40.
2. E.M. Kolibianakis, C. Albano, M. Camus, et al., "Prolongation of the Follicular Phase in in Vitro Fertilization Results in a Lower Ongoing Pregnancy Rate in Cycles Stimulated with Recombinant Follicle-Stimulating Hormone and Gonadotropinreleasing Hormone Antagonists," *Fertility and Sterility* 82 (2004): 102–7.
3. A. Seyhan, B. Ata, M. Polat, W.Y. Son, H. Yarali, and M.H. Dahan, "Severe Early Ovarian Hyperstimulation Syndrome Following GnRH Agonist Trigger with the Addition of 1500 IU hCG," *Human Reproduction* 28(9) (2013): 2522–8.
4. H.M. Fatemi, B. Popovic-Todorovic, P. Humaidan, S. Kol, M. Banker, P. Devroey, and J.A. García-Velasco, "Severe Ovarian Hyperstimulation Syndrome After Gonadotropin-Releasing Hormone (GnRH) Agonist Trigger and 'Freeze-All' Approach in GnRH Antagonist Protocol," *Fertility and Sterility* 101(4) (2014): 1008–11.
5. P. Humaidan, H. Ejdrup Bredkjaer, L.G. Westergaard, and C. Yding Andersen, "1500 IU Human Chorionic Gonadotropin Administered at Oocyte Retrieval Rescues the Luteal Phase When Gonadotropin-Releasing Hormone Agonist Is Used for Ovulation Induction: A Prospective, Randomized, Controlled Study," *Fertility and Sterility* 93 (2010): 847–54.
6. K.H. Lee, C.H. Kim, H.J. Suk, Y.J. Lee, S.K. Kwon, S.H. Kim, H.D. Chae, and B.M. Kang, "The Effect of Aromatase Inhibitor Letrozole Incorporated in Gonadotrophin Releasing Hormone Antagonist Multiple Dose Protocol in Poor Responders Undergoing in Vitro Fertilization," *Obstetrics & Gynecology Science* 57(3) (2014): 216–22.
7. A.J. DiLuigi, L. Engmann, D.W. Schmidt, C.A. Benadiva, and J.C. Nulsen, "A Randomized Trial of Microdose Leuprolide Acetate Protocol Versus Luteal Phase Ganirelix Protocol in Predicted Poor Responders," *Fertility and Sterility* 95(8) (2011): 2531–3.

57

Minimal Stimulation for IVF

Ippokratis Sarris and Geeta Nargund

Key Aspects of Mild Stimulation IVF

- Ovarian stimulation for IVF in a natural cycle using lower doses (lower daily dose and fewer days) of exogenous gonadotropins in comparison to down regulation followed by conventional stimulation.
- GnRH antagonist protocol instead of GnRH agonist protocol.
- Use of oral compounds (like anti-estrogens, or aromatase inhibitors) for ovarian stimulation either alone or in combination with exogenous gonadotropins.
- The aim is to achieve a mild response and higher "quality and not quantity" of oocytes.
- The aim is to prevent ovarian hyperstimulation syndrome (OHSS) with an ability to use GnRH agonist as a trigger if necessary.

Advantages of Mild Stimulation IVF

- Shorter treatment time
- Fitted in a woman's natural cycle
- Less expensive
- Less patient discomfort
- Safer, especially in the context of reducing the risk of OHSS and reducing potential long-term health implications to women and their children compared to conventional stimulation IVF due to the exposure to unphysiologically high levels of estrogen with the latter
- Potentially better oocyte, embryo, and endometrial quality
- Women's preference towards milder and safer approaches
- Widens access to treatment

Required Patient Information

- Age
- Anti-Müllerian hormone (AMH) level
- Antral follicle count (AFC 2–6 mm)
- Body mass index (BMI)
- History of previous stimulated cycles (if any):
  - Type of cycle
  - Dose and type of gonadotropin stimulation given (daily dose and duration)
  - Response—estradiol level on day of trigger, number of follicles above 12 mm, number of mature and immature eggs retrieved, fertilization rate, and embryo quality
- Complications

Choosing Type of Cycle, Stimulation Medication and Dose

- There is no single protocol or dosing algorithm, as what is important is to achieve a mild ovarian response with the lowest burden of medication and shortest duration.
- The aim is to use a lower cumulative dose of gonadotropins, which is achieved by either a late start of stimulation or by starting on a lower dose.
- The purpose of the former is to restrict ovarian stimulation to the mid- to late-follicular phase, permitting only few follicles to continue their development and therefore keeping the cycle as close as possible to the normal ovarian physiology.
- A number of protocols have been proposed:
  - Start a daily dose of 100–150 IU FSH on cycle day 2, along with GnRH antagonist fixed start (e.g., cycle day 6–7) or flexible start (when the lead follicle is 13 mm and/or the serum estradiol level is above 1000 pmol/L, with an endometrial thickness more than 5.5 mm with a triple layer appearance).

- Start a daily dose of 150 IU FSH once follicular dominance has developed (e.g., day 4–6) along with GnRH antagonist (with flexible start).
- Start oral compounds like anti-estrogens (such as clomiphene citrate or tamoxifen) or aromatase inhibitors (such as letrozole) on cycle day 2–3. These can either be stopped after 5 days and then continue with a daily low dose of FSH along and a GnRH antagonist with flexible start, or they can be continued up until the leading follicles are ready for trigger (with or without 2–3 alternate day "add-back" doses of 150 IU FSH).
- Luteal support is no different from the standard.
- Oral indomethacin can be used to prevent premature rupture of follicles if this is considered to be a risk.

Monitoring During Cycle

- Ultrasound evaluation prior to starting ovarian stimulation drugs to exclude the presence of cysts.
- Blood tests for serum estradiol and LH levels are useful.
- Urine LH testing can be used as an alternative to serum LH testing to monitor for a premature LH surge in cycles where oral compounds are used without GnRH antagonist.
- Indications for deciding on the timing of trigger can be the same as in conventional IVF, unless higher LH levels are detected in cycles without the use of GnRH antagonist.
- GnRH agonist is a trigger in women at risk of severe OHSS.

Disadvantages of Mild Stimulation IVF

- Difficulty in programming cycles and avoiding weekend oocyte retrievals.
- Embryology laboratory performance has to be excellent to be able to perform mild stimulation IVF effectively, as the smaller number of oocytes allows limited margin for errors.

- Smaller number of embryos are available for cryopreservation.
- There is a potential clinician "learning curve" when switching from conventional IVF to mild stimulation.

BIBLIOGRAPHY

Baart, E.B., E. Martini, M.J. Eijkemans, D. Van Opstal, N.G. Beckers, A. Verhoeff, N.S. Macklon, and B.C. Fauser. 2007. "Milder Ovarian Stimulation for in-Vitro Fertilization Reduces Aneuploidy in the Human Preimplantation Embryo: A Randomized Controlled Trial." *Human Reproduction* 22: 980–8.

Fauser, B.C.J.M., G. Nargund, A.N. Andersen, R. Norman, B. Tarlatzis, J. Boivin, and W. Ledger. 2010. "Mild Ovarian Stimulation for IVF: 10 Years Later." *Human Reproduction* 25: 2678–84.

Kwan, I., S. Bhattacharya, A. Kang, and A. Woolner. 2014. "Monitoring of Stimulated Cycles in Assisted Reproduction (IVF and ICSI)." *Cochrane Database of Systematic Reviews* 8: CD005289.

Nargund, G., B.C.J.M. Fauser, N.S. Macklon, W. Ombelet, K. Nygren, and R. Frydman. 2007. "Rotterdam ISMAAR Consensus Group on Terminology for Ovarian Stimulation for IVF. The ISMAAR Proposal on Terminology for Ovarian Stimulation for IVF." *Human Reproduction* 22(11): 2801–4.

Pelinck, M.J., M. Hadders-Algra, M.L. Haadsma, W.L. Nijhuis, S.M. Kiewiet, A. Hoek, M.J. Heineman, and K.J. Middelburg. 2010. "Is the Birthweight of Singletons Born After IVF Reduced by Ovarian Stimulation or by IVF Laboratory Procedures?" *RBM Online* 21: 245–51.

Revelli, A., A. Chiadò, P. Dalmasso, V. Stabile, F. Evangelista, G. Basso, and C. Benedetto. 2014. "'Mild' vs. 'Long' Protocol for Controlled Ovarian Hyperstimulation in Patients with Expected Poor Ovarian Responsiveness Undergoing in Vitro Fertilization (IVF): A Large Prospective Randomized Trial." *Journal of Assisted Reproduction and Genetics* 31: 809–15.

Verberg, M.F.G., M.J.C. Eijkemans, N.S. Machlon, E.M.E.W. Heijnen, E.B. Baart, F.P. Hohmann, B.C.J.M. Fauser, and F.J. Broekmans. 2009. "The Clinical Significance of the Retrieval of a Low Number of Oocytes Following Mild Ovarian Stimulation for IVF: A Meta-analysis." *Human Reproduction Update* 15: 5–12.

58

Ovarian Hyperstimulation Syndrome

Magued Adel Mikhail, Daniel Antonious, Candice P. Holliday, and Botros Rizk

Introduction

Ovarian hyperstimulation syndrome (OHSS) is the most serious complication of ovulation hyperstimulation. It is a systemic disease resulting from vasoactive products released by the hyperstimulated ovaries. Severe manifestations include thrombosis, renal and liver dysfunction, acute respiratory distress syndrome (ARDS), and rarely, death.

Pathophysiology of OHSS

OHSS is characterized by bilateral ovarian multi-cystic enlargement, ascites and third space fluid shift. The ovaries have significant stromal edema, theca-lutein cysts, and areas of cortical necrosis and neovascularization. The fluid shift is because of increased capillary permeability and fluid leakage mediated by vasoactive agents like vascular endothelial growth factor (VEGF).

Classification of OHSS

- OHSS can be classified depending on the onset into early and late onset.
  - Early OHSS presents 3 to 7 days after HCG and relates to excessive response to stimulation.
  - Late OHSS presents 12 to 17 days after HCG. It depends on pregnancy and is likely to be severe.
- OHSS can be classified, depending on severity, as mild, moderate and severe.
  - Mild: The mild degree was omitted from the new classification by Rizk and Aboulghar as it does not require any special treatment.
  - Moderate: Symptoms are abdominal pain, discomfort and distension. Hematological and biochemical profile are usually normal. There is no clinical evidence of ascites. Ultrasound reveals ascites and enlarged ovaries.
  - Severe:
    - Grade A: The symptoms include dyspnea, nausea, vomiting, abdominal pain, and oliguria. Clinically, there is marked abdominal distension and evidence of ascites. Hydrothorax can be evident on chest examination. Ultrasound show large ovaries and marked ascites. Hematological and biochemical profile can be abnormal.
    - Grade B: All of the criteria of Grade A plus severe dyspnea, massive tension ascites, marked oliguria, significantly enlarged ovaries, increased hematocrit, increased creatinine, and deranged liver function tests.
    - Grade C: Severity of Grade B complicated by respiratory distress, renal failure, or venous thrombosis.

The Incidence of OHSS

The estimated incidence of OHSS in IVF cycles is 20%–33% mild cases, 3%–6% moderate cases, and 0.1%–2% severe cases.

Prevention of OHSS

- Identifying the high-risk patients, monitoring cycles, coasting or delaying HCG, the use of GnRH agonist triggers, and cancelling the cycle are tools to prevent the occurrence of OHSS.
- Primary prevention aims to reduce the dose of gonadotropins and the "Ten Commandments" include identifying patients at risk, use of treatment of other than gonadotropins for PCOS patients—such as metformin and ovarian diathermy, and use of low doses and GnRH antagonists.
- Secondary prevention includes withholding or delaying hCG, follicular aspiration, cryopreservation of embryos, and progesterone for luteal phase support.

Management

- Other pathologies like ectopic pregnancy and ovarian torsion should be excluded.
- The management depends on severity, the presence of complications, and pregnancy.
- Management can be close monitoring, medical and surgical treatment.
- Electrolytic imbalance, hormonal and hemodynamic changes, pulmonary manifestation, liver dysfunction, hypoglobulinemia, neurological manifestations, adnexal torsion and thromboprophylaxis should be addressed.
- For moderate OHSS, the management is usually outpatient, with hospital admission if symptoms become severe.
- For severe OHSS Grade A, inpatient management is recommended unless the biochemical profile is normal and the patient is compliant with the outpatient management.
- For severe OHSS Grade B, the patients should have inpatient management with very close expert supervision.
- For severe OHSS Grade C, the patients should be treated in an intensive care setting.

Outpatient Management for Moderate OHSS

The management is mainly monitoring of symptoms, vital signs, biochemical profile, analgesia and thromboprophylaxis.

Inpatient Management for Severe OHSS

- Regular assessment of the vital signs, daily weight and girth measurement, and strict fluid balance, particularly urine output.
- Biochemical monitoring should include serum and electrolytes, renal and liver function tests, coagulation profile, and blood count.
- Ultrasonography can accurately assess the ovarian size and ascites and the location of pregnancy.
- Chest X-ray is needed if pleural effusion or hydrothorax is suspected.
- Respiratory or renal function deterioration requires blood gases and acid–base balance.
- Invasive hemodynamic monitoring like central venous pressure may be needed.

Medical Treatment

- The main aim is correction of the circulatory volume and the electrolyte imbalance by preserving adequate renal function.

- Volume replacement begins with intravenous crystalloid fluids at 125–150 mL/h.
- Plasma colloid expanders may be used. Albumin, dextran, mannitol, fresh frozen plasma, and hydroxyethyl starch (HAES) have also been used. If hypokalemia is significant, it should be corrected.
- Thromboprophylaxis with heparin or enoxaparin is mandatory. Anticoagulant therapy is indicated if there is clinical evidence of thromboembolic complications or laboratory evidence of hypercoagulability.
  - The duration of anticoagulation is debatable. It is recommended to continue during the first trimester of pregnancy. Some researchers suggest continuing until 20 weeks' gestation.
- Diuretic therapy without prior volume expansion can be detrimental, so should be restricted to the management of pulmonary edema.
- Dopamine in oliguric patients results in significant improvement in renal function.

Surgical Treatment

- Paracentesis offers temporary relief from respiratory and abdominal distress with reduction in the patient's weight, leg edema, and abdominal circumference. It also improves the urinary output. It is performed under ultrasonographic guidance to minimize the risk of injury to internal organs. Thoracocentesis may be necessary for patients with significant hydrothorax.
- There are several anesthetic challenges if surgery is needed, including thromboembolism tendency, hemoconcentration, pulmonary compromise, and ascites.
- Careful positioning is important, as the Trendelenburg position may further compromise the residual pulmonary functional capacity. IV access lines may be challenging.
- Laparotomy, in general, should be avoided in OHSS.
- In cases of hemorrhagic ovarian cysts, it should be performed by an experienced gynecologist to preserve the ovaries.
- In cases of ovarian torsion, only laparoscopic untwisting may be required, otherwise laparotomy is indicated.
- Surgical treatment for ectopic pregnancy is not commonly encountered.
- Pregnancy termination in extreme cases improves the clinical outcome of severe complications.

BIBLIOGRAPHY

Rizk, B. "Ovarian Hyperstimulation Syndrome." In *Progress in Obstetrics and Gynecology*, edited by J. Studd, 311–49. Edinburgh: Churchill Livingstone, 1993.

Rizk, B. *Ovarian Hyperstimulation Syndrome: Epidemiology, Pathophysiology, Prevention and Management.* Cambridge: Cambridge University Press, 2006.

Rizk, B. and M. Aboulghar. "Classification, Pathophysiology and Management of Ovarian Hyperstimulation Syndrome." In *A Textbook of In-vitro Fertilization and Assisted Reproduction*, 2nd ed., edited by P. Brinsden, 131–55. Carnforth: The Parthenon Publishing Group, 1999.

Rizk, B., and M. Aboulghar. "Ovarian Hyperstimulation Syndrome." In *Ovarian Stimulation*, edited by M. Aboulghar and B. Risk, 103–29. Cambridge: Cambridge University Press, 2011.

Rizk, B., and J. Smitz. 1992. "Ovarian Hyperstimulation Syndrome After Superovulation using GnRH agonists for IVF and Related Procedures." *Human Reproduction* 7(3): 320 –7.

Rizk, B., C.B. Rizk, M.G. Nawar, J.A. García-Velasco, and H.N. Sallam. "Ultrasonography in the Prediction and Management of Ovarian Hyperstimulationsyndome." In *Ulrasonography in Reproductive Medicine and Infertility*, edited by B. Rizk, 299–312. Cambridge: Cambridge University Press, 2010.

59

The Prediction of OHSS

Jan Gerris and Jana Claeys

Introduction

Ovarian hyperstimulation syndrome (OHSS) rarely occurs spontaneously in a natural cycle. The majority of cases are iatrogenic complications of so-called controlled ovarian hyperstimulation (COH) in women undergoing assisted reproductive technology (ART). It is a potentially life-threatening condition. The main symptoms are abdominal swelling and pain, breathing problems and oliguria. Hemo-concentration, ascites, deranged electrolyte parameters and generalized organ failure may occur. Thromboembolic events may also occur and fatal cases usually due to these have been reported.

OHSS is not uncommon. The most recent publications quote an incidence of 1%–5% in women treated with ART. Curently, clinical prognostic factors constitute the only possibility for prediction and prevention of OHSS.

Treatment is largely supportive; thus, it is crucial to prevent OHSS.

Pathophysiology

- The pathophysiology of OHSS is mostly due to an increase in vascular permeability, resulting in extravasation of intravascular fluid in the third space.
- The mechanism is the hCG-mediated increase in vascular endothelial growth factor (VEGF), an angiogenic cytokine that stimulates vascular endothelium. This can result either from exogenous hCG ("early OHSS") or from hCG produced by a successfully implanted embryo ("late OHSS").
- A genetic predisposition may play a role.

Risk Factors for OHSS (see Table 59.1)

- Identification of patients with a high risk of OHSS is imperative because treatment is largely supportive.
- Since embryo freezing has much improved using vitrification of blastocysts, the presence of one or more of these factors may constitute a reason for a segmented approach of treatment, i.e., freeze all oocytes retrieved and transfer frozen embryos one by one.
- Studies suggest that although no single parameter suffices to estimate the risk, the number of oocytes retrieved is likely to be the best indicator, because it is the most direct measure of ovarian response.
- Ten to twenty (or more) retrieved oocytes is the range that best predicts moderate to severe OHSS.
- This correlates with the number of intermediate sized follicles at the end of the stimulation.
- Given the correlation between high numbers of oocytes retrieved and the risk of OHSS, it seems reasonable to apply less aggressive stimulation protocols, especially in high responders.
- Using GnRH-agonists to trigger the ovulation in a GnRH-antagonist protocol may be an alternative for the use of hCG.

TABLE 59.1

Risk Factors Associated with OHSS

Primary Risk Factors
- Young age
- Lean body habitus
- PCOS (polycystic ovarian syndrome)
- High AMH levels (anti-Müllerian hormone)
- High antral follicle count (AFC)
- History of elevated response to gonadotropins

Secondary Risk Factors
- High-dose gonadotropin treatment
- High number of developing follicles and oocytes retrieved in ART cycles
- High serum estradiol (E2) levels on the day of ovulation triggering
- The need for coasting during COS
- Luteal phase hCG supplementation
- Pregnancy

BIBLIOGRAPHY

Aljawoan, F., L. Hunt, and U. Gordon. 2012. "Prediction of Ovarian Hyperstimulation Syndrome in Coasted Patients in an IVF/ICSI Program." *Journal of Human Reproductive Sciences* 5: 32–6.

Humaidan, P., J. Quartorolo, and E. Papanikolaou. 2010. "Preventing Ovarian Hyperstimulation Syndrome: Guidance for the Clinician." *Fertility and Sterility* 94: 389–400.

Kahnberg, A., A. Enskog, M. Brännström, K. Lundin, and C. Bergh. 2009. "Prediction of Ovarian Hyperstimulation Syndrome in Women Undergoing in Vitro Fertilization." *Acta Obstetricia et Gynecologica* 88: 1373–81.

Papanikolaou, E., P. Humaidan, N. Polyzos, and B. Tarlatzis. 2010. "Identification of the High-Risk Patient for Ovarian Hyperstimulation Syndrome." *Seminars in Reproductive Medicine* 28: 458–62.

Steward, R., L. Lan, A. Shah, J. Yeh, T. Price, J. Goldfarb, and S. Muasher. 2014. "Oocyte Number as a Predictor for Ovarian Hyperstimulation Syndrome and Live Birth: An Analysis of 256,381 in Vitro Fertilization Cycles." *Fertility and Sterility* 101: 967–73.

60

Tips on Technique of Embryo Transfer

Omar Abuzeid and Mostafa Abuzeid

Introduction

Successful outcome after in vitro fertilization-embryo transfer (IVF-ET) depends on embryo quality, endometrial receptivity, and the technique of embryo transfer. Meticulous and atraumatic transfer procedure is essential for a successful outcome.[1] Several factors have been shown to affect the success of ET:

- Cervical mucus[2]
- Blood
- Uterine contractions
- Proper delivery of embryos inside the uterine cavity[3]

In this chapter, we briefly discuss the principles for optimizing chances of successful ET. Special emphasis will be placed on:

- The role of ultrasound scan prior to and during ET procedure[4]
- Some practical points regarding ET techniques

A Problematic Cervix[5]

- Cervical problems are one of the most important factors that interfere with proper delivery of embryos inside the uterine cavity.
- Causes for cervical distortions:
  - Usually congenital in nature.
  - Sometimes as a result of cervical fibroid.
  - Rarely, as a result of a large Nabothian follicle or multiple Nabothian follicles.
- Causes of distortion in the utero-cervical angle:
  - Acutely anteverted/anteflexed uterus.
  - Retroverted uterus (especially, if the uterus is retroverted and fixed secondary to pelvic adhesions).
  - Extensive pelvic adhesions, leading to tilting of the uterus to one side, i.e., laterally.
  - When the uterus is tilted to one side, leading to an unusual lateral angulation as in patients with unicornuate uterus, especially in association with endometriosis and pelvic adhesions.
  - In rare cases, the utero-cervical angle may have the shape of almost a half-circle appearance for no obvious reason.
  - Some patients who underwent cesarean section (CS) may have an acute angle between the cervical canal and the lower uterine segment. This may be secondary to the healed CS scar pulling on and distorting this area.
  - Others may occasionally have a distorted angle as a result of adhesions between the uterus and the anterior abdominal wall.
- Other causes of problematic cervix:
  - The cervix may also be high in position after CS, or as a result of uterine fibroid or pelvic adhesions.
  - Sometimes the difficulty is due to narrowed external os; thus, the outer catheter is difficult to advance.
  - Sometimes the cervix is very short and flush with the lateral fornix (history of cone biopsy).
  - Cervical stenosis is a rare cause of difficult transfer (history of cone biopsy).
  - A cervical polyp may also interfere with ET procedure.

Assessment and Procedures prior to the Planned IVF-ET

- Include:
  - Careful history and physical examination.
  - Transvaginal ultrasound scan (2D and 3D).
  - Saline infusion sonohysterogram (2D and 3D).
- Certain correctable pathologies, including any causes of problematic cervix, that may interfere with implantation need to be identified and corrected surgically:
  - Submucosal fibroid.

- Endometrial polyps.
- Intrauterine scar tissue.
- Uterine septum.
- Mock trial catheter should be performed under ultrasound guidance.
- When a problematic cervix is identified, a plan of action needs to be formulated:
  - Consider cervical dilation and hysteroscopy.
  - In some patients hysteroscopy and resection of a ridge may be required. In this case, some investigators suggest leaving a Foley catheter in utero for one week after such procedures.
  - Consider cervical suture on day of oocyte retrieval or two days before ET in frozen thawed cycles.
  - Consider ET under transvaginal ultrasound scan guidance.
  - Use a special embryo transfer catheter that is meant for difficult transfer such as Rocket ET catheter (Rocket Medical PLC, Washington, England).
- If a mock trial is impossible and in the presence of at least one patent and healthy fallopian tube, consider tubal transfer procedure such as tubal embryo transfer on day 2 (TET).

Steps at Time of IVF-ET

- Valium 10 mg and Motrin 600 mg orally 30 minutes prior to ET.
- Use of transabdominal ultrasound scan helps in making ET procedure easy and atraumatic.
- Bladder filling should be optimum, avoiding under-distended or overdistended.
- Occasionally, fluid is seen in the endometrial cavity, which can be aspirated using embryo transfer catheter.
- Careful removal of cervical mucus through gentle suction and gentle irrigation using flushing media using a neonatal nasogastric tube (C. R. Bard, Inc. Covington, GA, USA).
- Avoid any trauma to the cervix that may result in bleeding as blood is associated with poor pregnancy rate.
- Avoid technique that may initiate uterine contractions during ET, such as grasping of the cervix with a tenaculum, touching the uterine fundus with the tip of the catheter, or passage of the outer rigid sheath of the ET catheter through the internal os.
- Mock trial should be done immediately before the actual ET.

- If the cervix is high in position, one cannot use a short catheter (18 mm); instead, use a 23 mm catheter.
- Meticulous ET should ensure proper delivery of embryos inside the uterine cavity.
- Ultrasound guidance allows the clinician to visualize the tip of the catheter.
- Embryos should be delivered gently about 1 cm from the fundal area.
- Embryologist should check the catheter to ensure that embryos are not present in the catheter.

Key Points in Clinical Practice

- Transvaginal ultrasound is mandatory for evaluation of the uterus and endocervical canal prior to and on the day of oocyte retrieval.
- Transabdominal ultrasound guidance is essential for meticulous and atraumatic ET.
- Cervical suture should be considered in patients with:
  - History of difficult mock trial.
  - History of problematic cervix.
  - History of pelvic adhesions (previous cesarean section).
  - Obesity.
- If severe difficulty is expected, consider:
  - Transvaginal ultrasound of ET.
  - Tubal embryo transfer, if possible.

REFERENCES

1. R.T. Mansour and M.A. Aboulghar, "Optimizing the Embryo Transfer Technique," *Human Reproduction* 17(5) (2002): 1149–53.
2. R.T. Mansour, M.A. Aboulghar, G.I. Serour, and Y.M. Amin, "Dummy Embryo Transfer Using Methylene Blue Dye," *Human Reproduction* 9 (1994): 1257–9.
3. H.N. Sallam, "Embryo Transfer Factors Involved in Optimizing the Success," *Current Opinion in Obstetrics and Gynecology* 17 (2005): 289–98.
4. A.M. Abou-Setta, "Effect of Passive Uterine Straightening During Embryo Transfer: A Systematic Review and Meta-Analysis," *Acta Obstetrica et Gynecologica* 86 (2007): 516–22.
5. M. Abuzeid and B. Rizk, "Ultrasonography-Guided Embryo Transfer," in *Ultrasonography in Reproductive Medicine and Infertility*, ed. B.R.M.B. Rizk. Cambridge: Cambridge University Press, 2010, 234–50.

61

Difficult Embryo Transfers

Gautam N. Allahbadia and Goral N. Gandhi

Factors of a Difficult Embryo Transfer (ET)

- It has been time-consuming
- The catheter met great resistance
- There was a need to change the catheter
- Sounding or cervical dilatation was needed
- A malleable stylet was required
- There was blood in any part of the catheter
- At least two attempts were required to successfully deposit the embryos

Required Equipment

- Ultrasound Unit with two probes; transvaginal and transabdominal
- Probe covers (non-latex, non-powdered)
- Ultrasound echogenic embryo transfer catheter
- Ultrasound echogenic trial embryo transfer catheter
- Embryo transfer malleable stylet
- Towako intramyometrial embryo transfer catheter set (in case of intramyometrial transfers)
- Culture media to flush endocervix
- Two mL syringe for flushing
- One mL syringe for ET
- Powder-free gloves
- Vulsellum
- Sponge-holding forceps
- Sponges
- Self-retaining bi-valve speculum
- Sims speculum
- Uterine sound
- One mm step dilator set

Preparation on the Day before ET

- Transfer media, flushing media and dishes are incubated overnight

Procedure: Transvaginal Sonography (TVS) Guided Embryo Transfer

- Generally done in patients with a retroverted uterus.
  1. A TVS examination of the uterus and pelvis is done *on an empty bladder* to confirm the size and position of the uterus, the direction and length of the utero-cervical canal, as well as the adnexae (to confirm no space-occupying masses that that might push the uterus away from its mid-posed position).
  2. A bi-valve self-retaining speculum is inserted into the vagina, bringing the external os to the center.
  3. Using a 2 mL syringe with pre-warmed flushing medium connected to an ultrasonic trial ET catheter, the catheter is advanced to the level of the external os. Without touching the tip of the catheter, forceful flushing of the external os is done, removing any cervical mucus present on the external os. Some mucus and secretions continue to fall over the posterior lip of the cervix with gravity. Do not use any sponge or cotton to remove any secretions—i.e., do not touch the cervix.
  4. Ultrasonic echogenic trial ET catheter is advanced to just beyond the internal os and removed to confirm the ease of transfer.
  5. Ultrasonic echogenic ET catheter loaded with embryos is now advanced under TVS guidance to the selected area of deposition of embryos, usually 1–1.5 cm from the fundus. In all the transfers, only 30 µL of transfer medium containing the embryos is gently expelled into the uterine cavity under TVS control. The catheter is gently removed immediately after transfer and then checked under a stereo microscope to ensure that all embryos have been transferred.
  6. In case of a "difficult" transfer, the Ultrasonic Echogenic soft ET catheter can be molded digitally to suit the curve of the utero-cervical canal.

Alternatively, a malleable stylet is used to guide the TVS transfer. Rarely, the Sims speculum and a vulsellum are needed to straighten the uterus. Even rarer is the use of uterine sounds and metal dilators.

Procedure: Transabdominal Sonography (TAS) Guided Embryo Transfer

- A TAS Guided transfer is the norm in all most units doing IVF.
  1. A bi-valve self-retaining speculum is inserted into the vagina, bringing the external os to the center.
  2. A TAS examination of the uterus and pelvis is done *on a partially full bladder* to confirm the size and position of the uterus, the direction and length of the utero-cervical canal, as well as the adnexae.
- The remainder of the procedure, Steps 3–6, are the same as detailed above in TVS, except using TAS, not TVS.

Procedure: TVS Intramyometrial Delivery into Uterine Cavity

- In rare cases of cervical agenesis or a mutilated cervix due to previous surgery or disease, a direct intramyometrial ET into the endometrial cavity using TVS guidance under short general anesthesia is required.
- Specialized intramyometrial transfer sets are available commercially for TVS guided intramyometrial transfers, which include a 17G 33 cm needle and a 40 cm ultrasoft ET catheter.
  1. A TVS examination of the uterus and pelvis is done *on an empty bladder* to confirm the size and position of the uterus, the direction and length of the utero-cervical canal, and the adnexae (for any space-occupying masses that might push the uterus away from its midposed position).
  2. The 17G 33 cm needle is advanced through the myometrium under TVS control until the tip reaches the central endometrial stripe. The ultrasoft ET catheter is threaded through the lumen into the endometrial canal.
  3. Approximately 10 µL of transfer medium is injected to confirm the tip of the ET catheter is in the endometrial cavity and the needle is steadied.
  4. The catheter is pulled out under TVS control, next loaded with the embryos along with 30 µL of transfer medium and reinserted into the endometrial cavity through the lumen of the needle.
  5. The transfer medium, containing the embryos, is gently expelled into the uterine cavity under TVS control.
  6. The catheter is gently removed immediately after transfer and checked under a stereo microscope to ensure that all embryos have been transferred.
  7. Once the expulsion is confirmed, the needle along with the catheter is removed.

Procedure: TAS Guided Intramyometrial Transfer Delivery into Uterine Cavity

- In rare cases of cervical agenesis or a mutilated cervix due to previous surgery or disease, direct intramyometrial ET into the endometrial cavity using TAS guidance under short general anesthesia is required.
- For TAS guided intramyometrial transfers, 16G or 17G amniocentesis needles and ultrasoft 40 cm ET catheters from commercially available GIFT sets are used.
  1. TAS examination of the uterus and pelvis is done *on an empty bladder* to confirm the size and position of the uterus, the direction and length of the utero-cervical canal, and the adnexae (for any space-occupying masses that might push the uterus away from its midposed position).
  2. The 16G 14 cm amniocentesis needle with an inner stylet is advanced transabdominally through the myometrium under TAS control until the tip reaches the central endometrial stripe. The inner metal stylet is removed and the ultrasoft ET catheter is threaded through the lumen into the endometrial canal.
- The remainder of the procedure, Steps 3–6, are the same as detailed above for TVS intramyometrial delivery into uterine cavity, except using TAS, not TVS.

BIBLIOGRAPHY

Akhtar, M.A., R. Netherton, K. Majumder, E. Edi-Osagie, and Y. Sajjad. 2015. "Methods Employed to Overcome Difficult Embryo Transfer During Assisted Reproduction Treatment." *Archives of Gynecology and Obstetrics* Feb 17. [Epub ahead of print] PubMed PMID: 25687658.

Phillips, J.A., W.P. Martins, C.O. Nastri, and N.J. Raine-Fenning. 2013. "Difficult Embryo Transfers or Blood on Catheter and Assisted Reproductive Outcomes: A Systematic Review and Meta-Analysis." *European Journal of Obstetrics & Gynecology and Reproductive Biology* 168(2): 121–8. doi: 10.1016/j.ejogrb.2012.12.030. Epub 2013 Jan 22.

Sullivan-Pyke, C.S., D.H. Kort, M.V. Sauer, and N.C. Douglas. 2014. "Successful Pregnancy Following Assisted Reproduction and Transmyometrial Embryo Transfer in a Patient with Anatomical Distortion of the Cervical Canal." *Systems Biology in Reproductive Medicine* 60(4): 234–8. doi: 10.3109/19396368.2014.917386. Epub 2014 May 5. PubMed PMID: 24797727.

Teixeira, D.M., L.A. Dassunção, C.V. Vieira, M.A. Barbosa, M.A. Coelho Neto, C.O. Nastri, and W.P. Martins. 2015. "Ultrasound Guidance During Embryo Transfer: A Systematic Review and Meta-Analysis of Randomized Controlled Trials." *Ultrasound in Obstetrics & Gynecology* 45(2): 139–48. doi: 10.1002/uog.14639. Epub 2015 Jan 5. PubMed PMID: 25052773.

62

In Vitro Maturation of Oocytes (IVM) for Fertility Treatment and Fertility Preservation

Michael H. Dahan, Justin Tan, Rabea Youcef Khoudja, Andrew Mok, and Seang Lin Tan

Introduction

- Indications for IVM:
  - To avoid ovarian hyperstimulation syndrome (OHSS) in women with high baseline follicle counts, i.e., PCO or PCOS.
  - For women who have a contraindication to ovarian stimulation, such as those with severe endometriosis which worsens with stimulation.
  - For women with current estrogen-sensitive malignancies.
- A baseline scan is performed day 2–3 of a spontaneous or progestin induced withdrawal bleed.
  - An endometrial lining >5 mm may suggest a previously missed polyp or fibroid, and a uterine evaluation should be undertaken if not recently done.
  - Moreover, since this procedure is often performed in women with PCOS, a thick lining after progestin withdrawal may represent an undiagnosed endometrial hyperplasia or malignancy. As such, endometrial sampling should be undertaken, particularly if the subject has a long history of anovulatory cycles and regular progestin withdrawal was not performed.
- At the time of the cycle day 2–3 scan, an evaluation of ovarian cysts and baseline follicle count should also be undertaken, since the baseline AFC gives a guide as to the number of oocytes which may be retrieved and the pregnancy rates.[1]
- Repeat scans are performed about 4–6 days later, when it is anticipated that a lead follicle of 10–14 mm in diameter may be obtained. This is because the retrieval of an *in vivo* matured oocyte will increase the pregnancy rate compared with retrieval of only GV oocytes.[2]
- Studies indicate that maximum pregnancy rates are obtained if the endometrium is at least 6–8 mm in maximum diameter with a triple line appearance on the day of oocyte collection.

HCG

IVM can be performed with or without triggering with HCG. However, we have found hCG trigger increases the number of MII oocytes obtained and the pregnancy rates.[3]

If 10,000 IU of HCG are given 38 hours before oocyte retrieval, the cumulous cells are fluffier, the number of oocytes collected is larger and more MII oocytes will be retrieved. Fluffier cumulous cells help the embryologist to locate the oocyte, particularly if they are less experienced at IVM. A sliding technique is used to help look for the oocytes.

It is a misconception to believe that MII oocytes are not collected from small follicles at IVM. Follicles as small as 4 mm in diameter have been known to yield MII oocytes. It appears that LH independent maturation of oocytes occurs in follicles that have initiated the pathway of atresia. Therefore, MII oocytes can be collected from small follicles. MII oocytes retrieved on the day of OPU yield embryos which have an equal potential for pregnancy, irrespective of the size of the follicles from which they are collected, i.e., < or >10 mm.

Timing of HCG

Ideally given when lead follicles are 10–14 mm in mean diameter and the endometrium is at least 6–8 mm maximum thickness with triple line. It is easier for less experienced doctors to retrieve oocytes from follicles above 10 mm and the likelihood of getting an *in vivo* matured oocyte is higher.

If the endometrium <6 mm maximum diameter, Estrace 12 mg (2 mg tid oral + 2 mg tid per vaginam) is given from the day of OPU. If endometrium is >8 mm, then Estrace 6 mg (2 mg tid oral) suffices. If Estrace is commenced before hCG trigger, follicular growth may be delayed.

If the follicles fail to grow to 10–12 mm, e.g., PCOS patient with anovulation, human menopausal gonadotropins 150 IU subcutaneous daily should be prescribed for 3–5 days, injection of which both thickens the endometrium and enlarges all the follicles.[4]

Egg collection is performed by using a 19 gauge single-lumen tapered needle. A reduced aspiration pressure as compared to in vitro fertilization egg collection is used

(12.0 kPa pr 90 cm Mercury). Multiple punctures are performed though the ovary. A recent advance has been the introduction of the Steiner-Tan IVM needle which has been shown to yield better results.[5]

A Pointer for Oocyte Collection

Since the needle is thinner and more likely to bend than an IVF needle and the smaller follicles can also be more difficult to puncture, hold the needle on the metal just prior to the connection with the plastic joint and not on the joint which is traditional with IVF collection. This will result in less bending of the needle. When in a follicle, rotate the needle, scraping the follicular walls, and stay in long after all the fluid is drained to help detach any adherent oocytes. The typical IVM egg collection lasts 20–30 minutes and on average 5–15 oocytes are obtained, although collection of up to 125 oocytes has been recorded.[6] Importantly, there is no greater incidence of complications or pain scores in IVM compared with IVF egg collections, and essentially no risk of OHSS.[7]

The embryologist performing IVM should be able to identify a germinal vesicle, MI and MII oocyte without stripping of the cumulus cells.

Any mature (MII) eggs are fertilized by ICSI 2–3 hours after oocyte collection.

If they are MI oocytes they are checked 12–16 hours after collection for conversion to an MII oocyte; germinal vesicle (GV) oocytes and MI are cultured in IVM media, several commercial brands are available. These media contain 75 IU of FSH and LH. Culture is performed for 24 to 48 hours. Oocytes are checked for maturity every 12 hours for up to 48 hours. Oocytes which remain GV after 24 hours but mature after 48 hours have a 90% chance of being genetically abnormal. Many centers culture for only 24 hours. As soon as the eggs reach MII stage, they are fertilized by ICSI. Embryo transfer is performed 2–5 days after ICSI.

To synchronize the endometrial lining for fresh transfer, estradiol valerate is administered from the day of OPU as 6 mg to 12 mg daily in divided doses. Progesterone support should also be commenced on the evening of oocyte collection in the same manner and dose as IVF.

Less common indications of IVM:

- Previous poor responders to ovarian stimulation—if maximum doses of FSH are given and very few eggs retrieved, IVM may be suitable if egg donation is declined.[8]
- Women who unexpectedly produce mostly poor-quality embryos with previous IVF at a young age.[9] Repeated pregnancy and live birth can be obtained by this method.
- Egg donation in women who are happy to donate eggs but are not keen to have ovarian stimulation.
- PGS or PGD cases in women who prefer to avoid ovarian stimulation.
- IVM fertility preservation in women to undergo chemotherapy for cancer treatment when there is no more time for ovarian stimulation for IVF or there is

contra-indication to use hormonal stimulation (see further Rao et al.).[10]

Results and Outcome of IVM Pregnancies

Results of IVM have shown that the pregnancy rate can be as high as 50% in women up the age of 37. The rate of congenital malformation following IVM is similar to the rates for IVF or ICSI.[11] The aneuploidy rate is comparable in IVF and IVM derived embryos.[12]

New Developments

There is recent research into improving the success rates of combined IVM and oocyte vitrification by using L Carnitine supplementation. The final development is recent studies showing that if fresh ET is not performed in IVM and the embryos are transferred in an FERC cycle, their pregnancy rates are comparable with those of IVF.

REFERENCES

1. S.L. Tan, T.J. Child, B. Gulekli, "In-Vitro Maturation and Fertilization of Oocytes from Unstimulated Ovaries: Predicting the Number of Immature Oocytes Retrieved by Early Follicular Phase Ultasonography," *American Journal of Obstetrics & Gynecology* 186 (2002): 684–9.
2. W.Y. Son, J.T. Chung, B. Herrero, N. Dean, E. Demirtas, H. Holzer, S. Elizur, R.C. Chian, and S.L. Tan, "Selection of the Optimal Day for Oocyte Retrieval Based on the Diameter of the Dominant Follicle in hCG-primed In Vitro Maturation Cycles," *Human Reproduction* 23 (2008): 2680–5.
3. R.C. Chian, W.M. Buckett, T. Tulandi, and S.L. Tan, "Prospective Randomized Study of Human Chorionic Gonadotropin Priming Before Immature Oocyte Retrieval in Unstimulated Women with Polycystic Ovarian Syndrome," *Human Reproduction* 15 (2000): 165–70.
4. S.E. Elizur, W.Y. Son, R. Yap, Y. Gidoni, D. Levin, E. Demirtas, and S.L. Tan, "Comparison of Low-Dose Human Menopausal Gonadotropin and Micronized 17ß-Estradiol in in Vitro Maturation Cycles with Thin Endometrial Lining," *Fertility and Sterility* 92 (2009): 907–12.
5. B.I. Rose and D. Laky, "A Comparison of the Cook Single Lumen Immature Ovum IVM Needle to the Steiner-Tan Pseudo Double Lumen Flushing Needle for Oocyte Retrieval for IVM," *Journal of Assisted Reproduction and Genetics* 30(6) (2013): 855–60.
6. M.H. Dahan, B. Ata, R. Rosenberg, J.T. Chunh, W.Y. Son, and S.L. Tan, "Collection of 125 Oocytes in an in Vitro Maturation Cycle Using a New Oocyte Collection Technique," *Journal of Obstetrics and Gynaecology Canada* 36 (2014): 900–3.
7. A. Seyhan, B. Ata, W.Y. Son, M.H. Dahan, and S.L. Tan, "Comparison of Complication Rates and Pain Scores After Transvaginal Ultrasound-Guided Oocyte Pickup

Procedures for in Vitro Maturation and in Vitro Fertilization Cycles," *Fertility and Sterility* 101 (2014): 705–9.

8. B. Gulekli, T.J. Child, R.C. Chian, and S.L. Tan, "Immature Oocytes from Unstimulated Polycystic Ovaries: A New Source of Oocytes for Donation." *Reproductive Technologies* 10 (2001): 295–7.

9. M. Al-Sunaidi, T. Tulandi, H. Holzer, C. Sylvestre, N. Dean, R.C. Chian, and S.L. Tan, "Repeated Pregnancies and Live Births After in-Vitro Maturation Treatment (Case Report)," *Fertility and Sterility* 87 (2007): 1212.

10. G.D. Rao, R.C. Chian, W.S. Son, L. Gilbert, and S.L. Tan, "Fertility Preservation in Women Undergoing Cancer Treatment," *The Lancet* 363 (2004): 1829.

11. R.C. Chian, L. Gilbert, J.Y.J. Huang, E. Demirtas, H. Holzer, A. Benjamin, W.M. Buckett, T. Tulandi, and S.L. Tan, "Live Birth After Vitrification of in Vitro Matured Human Oocytes," *Fertility and Sterility* 91 (2009): 372–6.

12. X.Y. Zhang, B. Ata, W.Y. Son, W.M. Buckett, S.L. Tan, and A. Ao, "Chromosome Abnormality Rates in Human Embryos Obtained From in-Vitro Maturation and IVF Treatment Cycles," *Reproductive Biomedicine Online* 21 (2010): 552–9.

63

Complications and Outcome of IVF

Jan Gerris

Outcome Variables

There is no absolute international agreement on what is a risk and what is a complication.

- In its annual report, the IVF monitoring program of ESHRE published the classical outcome variables of IVF, ICSI and IUI with partner and donor sperm, as well as a number of complications.
- Since 2008, the latter has stopped, probably due to severe irregularities, inconsistencies and international differences in data collection, as well as differences in definition.
- Traditionally, outcome variables for a so-called "fresh" IVF attempt (including ovarian stimulation) have been:
  - Number of oocytes at oocyte pick-up (OPU).
  - Number of mature oocytes at OPU.
  - Number of normally fertilized zygotes on day 1 after OPU.
  - Number of embryos fit for either transfer or cryopreservation (either on day 2–3 or day 5 after OPU).
  - Number of positive HCGs.
  - Ongoing pregnancies (amniotic sacs with cardiac activity).
  - Live births.
- All of these can be expressed per started cycle, per OPU, or per embryo transfer.
- Moreover, post-implantation variables can be expressed per fresh attempt or, in a cumulative

way, including the augmented result of any embryo transferred after freezing and thawing.
- The percentage of healthy born singletons as the cumulative result of one oocyte retrieval has been considered the highest quality outcome variable.

Complications

Complications are listed in Table 63.1 and the measures to minimize them in Table 63.2.

BIBLIOGRAPHY

de Mouzon, J., V. Goossens, S. Bhattacharya, J.A. Castilla, A.P. Ferrarretti, V. Korsak, M. Kupka, K.G. Nygren, and A. Nyboe Andersen, and The European IVF-monitoring (EIM) Consortium, for the European Society of Human Reproduction and Embryology (ESHRE). 2012. "Assisted Reproductive Technology in Europe, 2007: Results Generated From European Registers by ESHRE." *Human Reproduction* 27: 954–66.

Gerris, J., F. Olivennes, and P. De Sutter (eds). *Assisted Reproductive Technologies: Quality and Safety.* London: Parthenon Publishing, 2004.

Kupka, M.S., A.P. Ferrarretti, J. de Mouzon, K. Erb, T. D'Hooghe, J.A. Castilla, C. Calhaz-Jorge, C. De Geyter, V. Goossens, and The European IVF-monitoring (EIM) Consortium, for the European Society of Human Reproduction and Embryology (ESHRE). 2014. "Assisted Reproductive Technology in Europe, 2010: Results Generated From European Registers by ESHRE." *Human Reproduction* 29: 2099–113.

TABLE 63.1

Complication (Outcome)	Zero Tolerance Levels	Realistic Lowest Tolerance Level
Multiple pregnancies	0.9% (physiological) 1.5%–2% monozygotic	<10%
Ovarian hyperstimulation syndrome	0.0% (extremely rare)	<0.5%
Bleeding at oocyte retrieval	0.0%	?
Infection after oocyte retrieval	0.0%	?
Congenital anomalies	~ natural conception (3%–4%)	~ natural conception (3%–4%)
Cytogenetic abnormalities	~ natural conception (5%–6%)	~ natural conception (5%–6%)
Effects of cryopreservation	None	?
Effects of vitrification	None	?
Oncological effects	None	Probably none
Maternal deaths	None	Unrelated to ART
Fetal reduction	None	?
Psychosocial effects	None	None
Future fertility of ART children	None	?
Laboratory errors	None	KPI

TABLE 63.2

Complication (Outcome)	Measures to Be Taken to Minimize Them
Multiple pregnancies	Judicious application of single embryo transfer Strictly adhere to national or professional guidelines or draw them if nonexistent
Ovarian hyperstimulation syndrome	Primary prevention Secondary prevention Adequate management
Bleeding at oocyte retrieval	Minimize the number of puncture sites of the vaginal wall by moving straight from one follicle to the next
Infection after oocyte retrieval	Prophylactic antibiotics in case of endometrioma or previous PID
Congenital anomalies	Scrupulous follow-up of all ART pregnancies to screen and detect for anomalies
Cytogenetic abnormalities	Non-invasive prenatal testing whenever indicated
Effects of cryopreservation	Repeat analysis of well-documented long-term observational data on children born after cryopreservation and thawing of embryos
Effects of vitrification	Repeat analysis of well-documented long-term observational data on children born after vitrification and thawing of embryos
Oncological effects	Repeat analysis of well-documented long-term observational data on ART children
Maternal deaths	Optimize early pregnancy follow-up
Fetal reduction	Prevention by judicious embryo transfer policy
Psychosocial effects	Have risky or anxious patients screened by a reproductive psychologist
Future fertility of ART children	Long-term documentation of fertility issues in ART children, especially born after TESE+ICSI
Laboratory errors	Strictly adhere to a validates system of quality control based on critical performance indicators (CPIs)

64

Obstetric Complications after In Vitro Fertilization

Brian Brocato and David F. Lewis

Maternal Morbidities

Preterm Delivery

Preventative Measures

- No prior history of spontaneous preterm delivery:
  - Cervical length (CL) between 16 and 20 weeks' gestation.
  - Vaginal progesterone if CL <20 mm.[1]
- Prior history of spontaneous preterm delivery:
  - Weekly intramuscular 17 alpha hydroxyprogesterone caproate beginning from 16 weeks' gestation through 36 weeks' gestation.[2]
  - Consider serial CL surveillance in women with prior delivery before 34 weeks' gestation. Consider cerclage if CL less than 15 mm between 16 and 24 weeks' gestation.[3]
- Educate and screen for signs and symptoms of preterm delivery during prenatal visits.
- Preventative measures such as cerclage, bedrest, pessary, and prophylactic tocolytics have not been shown beneficial in multiple gestations.[4]

Management of Threatened Preterm Labor

- Observation on labor and delivery unit
- Consider tocolysis if evidence of labor with cervical change
- Corticosteroids between 22 and 34 weeks' gestation[5]
- Magnesium sulfate for neuroprotection if delivery considered imminent
- Group B *streptococcus* prophylaxis
- Delivery recommended in facility with appropriate resources to care for premature neonates

Preterm Premature Rupture of Membranes (PPROM)

- Diagnosis by history and physical exam (presence of pooling of amniotic fluid, ferning of dried amniotic fluid under microscope, nitrazine test of amniotic fluid)
- Treated expectantly inpatient between 22 and 34 weeks' gestation
- Corticosteroids between 22 and 34 weeks' gestation
- Antibiotics for latency (amoxicillin and erythromycin) for 1 week
- Magnesium sulfate for neuroprotection if delivery considered imminent
- Daily antepartum testing
- Delivery is indicated if evidence of labor, chorioamnionitis or non-reassuring fetal testing
- Delivery at 34 weeks' gestation in the absence of other indications

Preeclampsia

Prevention

- Women with a history of early onset preeclampsia or preeclampsia in more than one prior pregnancy
- Low-dose aspirin beginning in the late first trimester[6]
- Educate and screen for signs and symptoms of preeclampsia

Management of Hypertensive Disorders of Pregnancy

- Consult Maternal-Fetal Medicine to determine optimal management and delivery plan.
- Assess for severe features of preeclampsia.
- Screen for HELLP syndrome—CBC, chemistry, liver function.
- Magnesium sulfate to prevent eclampsia if meets severe criteria.
- Control maternal blood pressure with intravenous antihypertensive agents (first-line agents labetalol or hydralazine).
- Corticosteroids between the gestational ages of 22–34 weeks.

- Mild disease can be managed until 37 weeks' gestation.

Placenta Previa

- Assess placental location in the second trimester, at the time of the fetal anatomy survey.
- If previa diagnosed, pelvic rest and bleeding precautions.
- Delivery recommended between 34 and 36 weeks' gestation.

Fetal Morbidities

Congenital Anomalies

- Offer serum analyte screening for aneuploidy and open spina bifida.
- Screen for fetal anomalies at 18–20 weeks' gestation.
- Fetal echocardiogram at 22 weeks' gestation.[7]

Fetal Demise

- Consider antenatal testing beginning at 32 weeks' gestation.[8]

Fetal Growth Restriction

- Measure fundal height at each prenatal visit.
- Consider ultrasound for fetal growth assessment at 28–32 weeks' gestation.
- Serial ultrasounds to assess fetal growth every 3–4 weeks if additional risk factor for fetal growth restriction.
- Refer to Maternal-Fetal-Medicine if overall estimated fetal weight <10th percentile or abdominal circumference <5th percentile.[9]
- Once growth restriction diagnosed, begin antenatal testing and umbilical artery Doppler studies.

Prenatal Care

- Routine prenatal care is recommended.
- Screen for comorbidities such as obesity, advanced maternal age and other chronic medical conditions (diabetes, hypertension, thyroid abnormalities) that may impact pregnancy outcome.
- Maternal serum analyte screening for aneuploidy may be altered in women undergoing assisted reproductive technology.[10]

Labor and Delivery

- In the absence of other indications, delivery at term.
- Cesarean delivery reserved for obstetric indications only.

REFERENCES

1. S.S. Hassan, R. Romero, D. Vidyadhari, S. Fusey, J.K. Baxter, M. Khandelwal, et al., "Vaginal Progesterone Reduces the Rate of Preterm Birth in Women with a Sonographic Short Cervix: A Multicenter, Randomized, Double-Blind, Placebo-Controlled Trial," *Ultrasound in Obstetrics & Gynecology* 38(1) (2011): 18–31.
2. P.J. Meis, M. Klebanoff, E. Thom, M.P. Dombrowski, B. Sibai, A.H. Moawad, et al., "Prevention of Recurrent Preterm Delivery by 17 Alpha-Hydroxyprogesterone Caproate," *New England Journal of Medicine* 348(24) (2003): 2379–85.
3. J. Owen, G. Hankins, J.D. Iams, V. Berghella, J.S. Sheffield, A. Perez-Delboy, et al., "Multicenter Randomized Trial of Cerclage for Preterm Birth Prevention in High-Risk Women with Shortened Midtrimester Cervical Length," *American Journal of Obstetrics and Gynecology* 201(4) (2009): 375 e1–8.
4. American College of Obstetricians and Gynecologists Committee on Practice Bulletins-Obstetrics, Society for Maternal-Fetal Medicine, and ACOG Joint Editorial Committee, "ACOG Practice Bulletin #56: Multiple Gestation: Complicated Twin, Triplet, And High-Order Multifetal Pregnancy," *Obstetrics and Gynecology* 104(4) (2004): 869–83.
5. T.N. Raju, B.M. Mercer, D.J. Burchfield, and G.F. Joseph, Jr., "Periviable Birth: Executive Summary of a Joint Workshop by the Eunice Kennedy Shriver National Institute of Child Health and Human Development, Society for Maternal-Fetal Medicine, American Academy of Pediatrics, and American College of Obstetricians and Gynecologists," *American Journal of Obstetrics and Gynecology* 210(5) (2014): 406–17.
6. American College of Obstetricians and Gynecologists, *Task Force on Hypertension in Pregnancy, American College of Obstetricians and Gynecologists. Hypertension in Pregnancy*. Washington, DC: American College of Obstetricians and Gynecologists, 2013.
7. American Institute of Ultrasound in Medicine, "AIUM Practice Guideline for the Performance of Fetal Echocardiography," *Journal of Ultrasound in Medicine* 32(6) (2013): 1067–82.
8. Practice Bulletin No. 145: Antepartum Fetal Surveillance. *Obstetrics and Gynecology* 124(1) (2014): 182–92.
9. J.A. Copel and M.O. Bahtiyar, "A Practical Approach to Fetal Growth Restriction," *Obstetrics and Gynecology* 123(5) (2014): 1057–69.
10. S.T. Chasen, "Maternal Serum Analyte Screening for Fetal Aneuploidy," *Clinical Obstetrics and Gynecology* 57(1) (2014): 182–8.

65

Twins Pregnancy after ART

David F. Lewis and Brian Brocato

Ultrasound to Evaluate Twins[1]

- Determine type of twin (monozygotic/dizygotic)
- Determine chorionicity and amnionicity by 14 weeks:
  - Number of gestational sacs equals the number of chorions
  - Number of yolk sacs equals the number of amnions
- Assess adnexa

Discuss Prenatal Care[2]

- Weight gain targets
- Prenatal diagnosis technique—benefits and limitations
- Prenatal vitamins and supplements
- Increased risk for preterm delivery:
  - Preterm labor: 55%
  - Preterm premature rupture of membrane: 22%
  - Indicated deliveries for complications: 23%
- Increased risk of preeclampsia
- Increased risk for growth restriction and/or discordancy
- Increased risk of abruption
- Increased risk of previa
- Increased risk of fetal anomalies, including cardiac defects
- Increased maternal risks
- Detailed plan based on chorionicity and amnionicity
- Delivery plan—indications for cesarean delivery

First Trimester

- Complete history and physical
- Routine prenatal labs
- Start ASA 81 mg at 12 weeks[3]
- Blood pressure, urine dip
- Interval of visits at least every 4 weeks

Second Trimester

- Level 2 ultrasound with fetal echocardiography 18–22 weeks
- Start serial ultrasounds for growth every 4 weeks
- Preterm labor signs and symptoms discussed
- Preeclampsia signs and symptoms discussed
- Glucola 24–28 weeks
- Tdap administration

Third Trimester

- Serial ultrasound for growth every 4 weeks
- Visits every 2 weeks until 36 weeks, then weekly
- Plan for delivery based on fetal presentation and obstetrical complications
- Dichorionic twins delivery at 38 weeks in the absence of other indications

Delayed Delivery of Twin[4]

Delivery of First Twin

- If second twin does not delay, discuss risks with patient including:
  - Infection
  - Hemorrhage
  - DVT
  - Coagulation disorders
  - Death
- Fetal:
  - Extreme developmental delay
  - Cerebral palsy
  - Infection
  - Periventricular leukomalacia
- Delivery of placenta if cord not very high
- Consider antibiotics, cerclage and tocolysis depending on situation
- Watch closely for infection

- Consider steroids/magnesium sulfate for neuroprotection at viability
- Serial ultrasound for growth
- Antenatal testing

Death of One Twin

- Explain risk to patient at first visit. Higher risk, the earlier the gestational age. Monochorionic/monoamniotic is at greater risk than dichorionic/diamniotic
- Increased risk of losing surviving twin after 14 weeks
- Explain risk of neurological infection to surviving twin MC 18%, DC 1%
- At viability ≥23 weeks, but ≤34 weeks, expectant management
- Corticosteroids and magnesium sulfate for neuroprotection
- Antepartum testing
- Serial ultrasounds for growth every 3 to 4 weeks
- If death after 20 weeks, serial coagulation studies
- Delivery by 34 weeks

Monochorionic/Diamniotic Twins

- Establish diagnosis by 14 weeks
- Counsel patient:
  - Fetal anomalies
  - Risk of preterm birth, growth restriction, twin to twin transfusion syndrome (TTTS), postpartum hemorrhage—10% develop evidence of TTTS, assess bladder, fluid, cardiac function with Doppler plus assess stage:
    - Stage I and II, consider amnioreduction
    - Stage III and IV, to regular care for possible laser antepartum testing and close follow-up
    - Low threshold for referrals to Fetal Care Center
  - Fetal death of one twin with potential sequelae for surviving twin
  - Serial ultrasound at 16 weeks, every 2 weeks until 28 weeks. Evaluating for fetal bladder, growth, greatest vertical pocket around both twins
  - After 28 weeks, every 2 to 3 weeks and growth every 4 weeks
  - Detailed anatomic survey and fetal echo 18–22 weeks
  - Uncomplicated delivery by 37 6/7 weeks

Monochorionic/Monoamniotic[5]

- Establish EDC, chorionicity, amniocity by 14 weeks
- Counsel about risk of monochorionic/monoamniotic twins:
  - Congenital anomalies
  - Pregnancy complications:
    - Preterm birth
    - Growth restriction
    - TTTS
    - Postpartum hemorrhage
    - Fetal death of one twin with potential sequelae to surviving twin
    - Antepartum management including monitoring
    - Plan for delivery
- Management:
  - Ultrasounds every 2 weeks starting at 16 weeks to 28 weeks looking at bladders, amniotic fluid volume ≥28 weeks, every 2–3 weeks
  - Detailed anatomical survey/fetal echocardiogram 18–22 weeks
  - Elective cesarean section 32–34 weeks
- Other complications:
  - Preterm labor
  - Preterm premature rupture of membranes
  - Abruption

REFERENCES

1. American College of Obstetrics and Gynecology, Practice Bulletin No. 144. *Multifetal Gestations: Twin, Triplet, and Higher-Order Multifetal Pregnancies*. American College of Obstetrics and Gynecology, 2014, 1–8.
2. American Academy of Pediatrics, *Guidelines for Perinatal Care*, 7th ed. American College of Obstetrics and Gynecology, 2012.
3. M.L. LeFevre, "Low-Dose Aspirin Use for the Prevention of Morbidity and Mortality From Preeclampsia: U.S. Preventative Services Task Force," *Annals of Internal Medicine* 161 (2014): 819–26. doi:10.7326/M14–1884.
4. A. Rao, S. Sairam, and H. Shehata, "Obstetric Complications of Twin Pregnancies," *Best Practice & Research in Clinical Obstetrics and Gynecology* 18(4) (2004): 557–76.
5. L.L. Simpson, "Twin-Twin Transfusion Syndrome: Society for Maternal-Fetal Medicine," *American Journal of Obstetrics and Gynecology* 208 (2013): 3–18.

66

IVF and Endometriosis

Graciela Kohls Ilgner and Juan Antonio García-Velasco

Required Equipment

- Ultrasound scan

To Prepare before the Ovarian Stimulation

- Evaluate the location and sizes of the endometriomas by ultrasound scan.
- Determine the accessibility of the follicles during the oocyte pick-up (OPU).
- Check the mobility of the ovaries to reach the healthy ovarian tissue during the OPU.
- If the ovaries are fixed and the follicles are out of reach, consider the surgery.
- Check the ovarian reserve by antral follicle count (AFC), AMH or basal FSH and estradiol.
- Establish the ovarian protocol; most patients with endometriosis have low ovarian reserve.

GnRH Agonist Ultra-Long Protocol

- Use prolonged pituitary suppression of typically 3 cycles of GnRH agonist before stimulation begins. Alternatively, we may give 2 months of continuous OCP.
- This protocol has been shown to be particularly useful for patients with stage 3 or 4 endometriosis.

During the Ovarian Stimulation

- Check the fallopian tubes because some hydrosalpinges could appear during the ovarian stimulation.
- Patients with endometriosis have higher risk of hydrosalpinx.

Preparation before the OPU

- The risk of infection after OPU is as low as 0.3–0.6%.[1]
- We usually prescribe antibiotic (azithromycin p.o. 1 g) the night before OPU in all the patients.

During the OPU

- In patients with endometriomas the risk of infection is still low, but higher than in other patients.
- Thus, must consider IV antibiotics if an endometrioma was accidentally punctured during the procedure.[2]

During Embryo Transfer (ET)

- Antibiotic is not systematically used for ET, but in patients with high risk of tubo-ovarian abscess who did not receive prophylaxis the days before, should consider it.

Complications of Endometriosis

- Rupture of the endometrioma

Oocyte Quality or the Endometrium

- Pregnancy rates are decreased in endometriosis compared with tubal factor.
- The pathology (endometrium or oocyte negative impact) is still debated in the literature.

REFERENCES

1. J. Remohí, J. Bellver, J. Domingo, E. Bosch, and A. Pellicer, *Manual Práctico De Esterilidad Y Reproducción Humana*. Madrid: McGraw Hill, 2008, 285–93.
2. L. Benaglia, E. Somigliana, R. Iemmello, E. Colpi, A.E. Nicolosi, and G. Ragni, "Endometrioma and Oocyte Retrieval-Induced Pelvic Abscess: A Clinical Concern or an Exceptional Complication?" *Fertility and Sterility* 89 (2008): 1263–6.

67

Leiomyoma of the Uterus

Shawky Z.A. Badawy

Introduction

Leiomyomas are considered to be the most common benign tumors of the uterus. These leiomyomas could be present in the body of the uterus, cervical part of the uterus, or both locations. They have estrogen and progesterone receptors, and therefore they respond to ovarian hormones and continue to grow. The degree of growth could be slow or relatively high. Leiomyomas constitute a health problem for women because of frequent visits to the medical offices for treatment, recurrences, and fertility issues. It is also one of the most common causes of hysterectomy in the United States.

Pathophysiology

- The theories of how these leiomyomas develop include either from smooth muscle cells of the wall of the uterus or from smooth muscle cells surrounding the neighboring blood vessels.
- These smooth muscle cells are intermingled with fibrous tissue and the leiomyoma usually has a "false capsule," which is compressed tissue from the surrounding uterine wall.
- Thus during surgery, in order to reach the actual myoma to be removed, the surgeon has to open the capsule, clear the myoma, and then close the capsule again and it becomes part of the uterine wall.
- The blood supply to the myoma comes from branches and tributaries of the uterine vessels.
- With the enlargement of the myoma, the vascular supply increases and that will lead to the problems of heavy uterine bleeding, which is a common symptom.
- Uterine leiomyomas may undergo certain changes called degeneration, including hyaline degeneration, cystic degeneration. In this type of degeneration, the cells undergo hyalinization and then cystic changes in the form of cavities occur in these leiomyomas.
- Another type of degeneration is red degeneration, which might be due to certain hemorrhagic episodes

in the leiomyoma. This is especially present during pregnancy.
- If the leiomyoma is pedunculated, then there is a possibility of torsion of the myoma around its pedicle, and the blood supply is affected. This will lead to severe pain and requires emergency surgery.
- During pregnancy these leiomyomas usually increase in size due to the stimulation of the pregnancy hormones, especially the high levels of estrogen and progesterone. This may lead to miscarriages, premature deliveries, malpresentations, and an increase in cesarean section rates.

Clinical Picture

- Leiomyomas can be completely asymptomatic if they are small in size and either subserosal or intramural. Under these circumstances they need just a follow-up every six months in order to detect any early changes.
- The major symptom of uterine leiomyoma is uterine bleeding in the form of heavy menstrual flow, especially with submucosal and intramural myomas. This bleeding could be severe and may lead to anemia. In addition, such types of leiomyomas will lead to infertility, because of the poor endometrial environment that will interfere with implantation. Lastly, the pressure effect on the fallopian tubes, especially if the leiomyomas are intraligamental, interferes with the ovum pick-up and fertilization.
- Large leiomyomas in the body of the uterus or cervix will lead to pressure on the urinary bladder, leading to increased frequency of urination or difficulty in urination. Especially around the time of the menses, there will be marked edema and these patients will present to the office or emergency room with acute urinary retention.

Diagnosis

- Those patients who have enlarged uteri on pelvic exam and also have symptoms suggestive of leiomyomas need radiologic evaluation to define the size and location of the myoma to assist in the proper treatment.
- Ultrasound evaluation is usually the first step, which usually shows the location of the myoma and its size and helps in the treatment.
- MRI of the pelvis will not add much to the ultrasound evaluation, unless the ovaries cannot be clearly evaluated with the ultrasound.

Management of Leiomyomas

- For infertility cases, it is important to do a hysterosalpingogram to define the condition of the uterine cavity and fallopian tubes before any surgical intervention is carried out.
- Surgical intervention could be in the form of laparoscopy or laparotomy for intramural and subserosal myomas. For submucosal myomas, hysteroscopic resection is the standard.
- There have been many discussions recently about laparoscopic surgery and removal of the myoma from the abdominal cavity. It is agreed that these myomas should be intact without any morcellation that may lead to leaving pieces in the peritoneal cavity that might prove in the future to be malignant. This is why many centers in the United States suggest that the myoma should be removed intact, and have discontinued the morcellation practice.
- In very symptomatic patients who have completed their families and do not wish to achieve pregnancy, a hysterectomy would be the best choice. Of course, if the patient has not reached the menopausal age, then the ovaries could be left to support the body with the ovarian hormones that are important for the well-being of the individual.

New Management Options

- MRI-guided ultrasound waves:
  - Ultrasound waves can be directed toward the myoma via MRI pictures and to lead to shrinkage of the myoma over time.
  - This is a recent method, and more data is needed to evaluate the effectiveness of this technology.
- Uterine artery embolization (UAE):
  - UAE is a non-invasive, outpatient procedure by an interventional radiologist.
  - A catheter is introduced through the femoral artery, the iliac artery, and the uterine artery and then embolization is done to stop the blood flow to the myoma.
  - The myoma will gradually decrease in size and also the symptoms of bleeding will subside.
- GnRH agonists:
  - The use of GnRH agonists have been advocated, especially for pre-operative preparation of the patient.
  - Usually with the GnRH agonist the patients develops hypogonadotropic hypogonadism.
  - The fibroids then shrink in size in three months, usually with a degree of reduction of about 50%.
  - This technique has been shown to facilitate removal of myomas surgically with proper reconstruction of the uterus.
  - The side effects are vasomotor symptoms and some degree of bone loss.
  - The patient can be given a very small dose of a progestin during that treatment if needed to alleviate the symptoms of hot flashes.

BIBLIOGRAPHY

Evans, P. and S. Brunsell. 2007. "Uterine Fibroid Tumors: Diagnosis and Treatment." *American Family Physician* 75(10): 1503–8.

Manga, A.K., C.R. Woodhouse, and S.L. Stanton. 1996. "Pregnancy and Fibroids Causing Simultaneous Urinary Retention and Ureteric Obstruction." *British Journal of Urology* 77: 606–7.

Marino, J.L., B. Eskenazi, M. Warnder, S. Samuels, P. Vercellini, N. Gavoni, et al. 2004. "Uterine Leiomyoma and Menstrual Cycle Characteristics in a Population Based Cohort Study." *Human Reproduction* 19: 2350–5.

Myers, E.R., M.D. Barber, T. Gustilo-Ashby, G. Couchman, D.B. Matcher, and D.C. McCrory. 2002. "Management of Leiomyomata: What Do We Really Know?" *Obstetrics & Gynecology* 100: 8–17.

Schwartz, P.E., and M.G. Kelly. 2006. "Malignant Transformation of Myomas: Myth or Reality?" *Obstetrics & Gynecology Clinics of North America* 33: 183–98, xii.

Wilcox, L.S., L.M. Koonin, R. Pokras, L.T. Strauss, Z. Sia, and H.B. Peterson. 1994. "Hysterectomy in the United States, 1988–1990." *Obstetrics & Gynecology* 83: 549–55.

68

Office Management of Polycystic Ovarian Syndrome

Shawky Z.A. Badawy

Diagnostic Criteria for Polycystic Ovarian Syndrome (PCOS)

Two of the following three criteria must be met:

- Amenorrhea/oligomenorrhea and anovulation
- Hyperandrogenism and/or hyperandrogenemia
- Ultrasound appearance of polycystic ovaries

These patients will have irregular cycles, absent ovulation, and either elevated androgen levels or the presence of hirsutism.

Endocrine Studies

- Endocrine studies include the following: thyroid evaluation (using TSH and T4), prolactin level, cortisol level, dehydroepiandrostene sulfate and total and free testosterone levels.
- In the past, FSH and LH levels were ordered based on the fact that LH secretion is higher than FSH secretion because of the suppression of the hypothalamic pituitary factor with the high levels of circulating estrogens. This is not diagnostic, however, because it could be present in obese anovulatory patients who do not have polycystic ovarian syndrome.
- The main endocrine finding in patients with PCOS is elevated testosterone level; either the total and free levels or simply the free testosterone level would be in excess.
- The clinical presentation of these patients will include amenorrhea/oligomenorrhea, hirsutism, and infertility. We will focus our management after that on these clinical pictures.

Management of Amenorrhea/Oligomenorrhea

- Treatment of this symptomotology is essential in order to prevent uterine bleeding and to prevent endometrial changes that will lead to hyperplasia and cancer of the endometrium.

- Patients can be treated with the use of steroidal oral contraceptives.
  - These oral contraceptives will cycle the endometrium and prevent the occurrence of hyperplasia and cancer.
  - It will lead to regular cycles and patients will be comfortable anticipating the onset of their menstrual cycles on a regular basis.
  - Third-generation pills contain desogestrol as a progestin, which has a high affinity for progesterone receptors and does not attach itself to androgen receptors. Thus it is free of androgenecity.
  - Fourth-generation birth control pills containing drospirenone as a progestin can also be used. This has been proven to be very good in alleviating the symptoms of irregular cycles as well as the hirsutism.
- Ensure that there are no contraindications to the use of the pill.
  - If there is a contraindication to the use of the pill, then these patients could be prescribed progestins only in a cyclic fashion to be used 10 days every month.
  - This will prevent hyperplasia of the endometrium and lead to regular cycles during its use.
  - However, these cyclic progestins will not act as contraceptive, and therefore patients should use the barrier method to protect against occasional ovulation and pregnancy that could occur.
- These lines of treatment are very satisfactory for the teenage population as well as reproductive-age women who do not want to achieve pregnancy at the present time.

Treatment of Hirsutism

- Hirsutism results from the excess of androgens.

- As a result of that, there will be hair growth on the face, chest, abdomen in addition to excessive secretions and oily skin and perhaps acne.
- The treatment of such conditions is to use birth control pills.
- This usually takes at least six months for significant change to be noticeable by the patient.
- The patient should continue after that to maintain these changes.
- Sometimes the process is slow and the patient asks for other management, such as electrolysis or laser hair removal.

Treatment of Infertility

- The treatment is induction of ovulation.
- Before that step is taken, the treating physician has to be sure that the hysterosalpingogram is completed, and there are no uterine or tubal factors.
- In addition, the male factor also has to be evaluated.
- There are several agents that are used at the present time for induction of ovulation.

Clomiphene Citrate

- Clomiphene citrate is a SERM that leads to stimulation of folliculogenesis and steroidogenesis from the ovary.
- Around midcycle with the elevation of estradiol to a peak, that will stimulate the LH as the triggering hormone for maturation of the oocyte and ovulation.
- Clomiphene citrate is usually very successful in inducing ovulation in about 80% of patients.
- It is to be noted that with the high testosterone levels in these patients, clomiphene citrate might not be as effective as in patients who are simply anovulatory and not PCOS. For this reason, it is essential to lower the testosterone level in these patients. This could be accomplished either by putting the patient on birth control pills two cycles prior to starting the ovarian stimulation, or by putting the patient on Glucophage. Glucophage lowers insulin levels,

thus lowering testosterone level. The combination of metformin and clomiphene citrate might be helpful in such patients who failed to respond to clomiphene citrate alone.

Gonadotropins

- Purified urinary gonadotropins or recombinant gonadotropins have a higher success rate in induction of ovulation as compared to clomiphene citrate. However, the multiple pregnancy rate will be higher than with clomiphene citrate.
- It is important at this stage of treatment of PCOS to consult or to refer the patient to a reproductive endocrinologist because they have the facilities and time to follow up these patients closely.
- Ovarian drilling has been tried in PCOS patients. There are no clearly controlled studies to support it as a superior method to facilitate ovulation. Furthermore, studies show that this could lead to peritubal and periovarian adhesions that complicates the process.

BIBLIOGRAPHY

Amer, S.A., T.C. Li, and W.L. Ledger. 2004. "Ovulation Induction Using Laparoscopic Ovarian Drilling in Women with Polycystic Ovarian Syndrome. Predictors of Success." *Human Reproduction* 19: 1719–24.

Dunaif, A. 1997. "Insulin Resistance and the Polycystic Ovary Syndrome: Mechansim and Implications for Pathogenesis." *Endocrine Reviews* 18(6): 774–800.

Lord, J.M., I.H.K. Flight, and R.J. Norman. 2003. "Metformin in Polycystic Ovary Syndrome. Systemic Review and Meta Analysis." *BMJ* 327(7421): 951–3.

Roy, S., R.B. Greenblatt, D.R. Mahesh, Jr., E. Bailey. 1982. "A Decade's Experience with an Individualized Clomiphene Treatment Regimen Including Its Effect on the Post Coital Test." *Fertility and Sterility* 37: 161–7.

Stein, I.F., and M.L. Leventhal. 1935. "Amenorrhea Associated with Bilateral Polycystic Ovaries." *American Journal of Obstetrics & Gynecology* 29: 181–91.

Yildz, BO. 2008. "Oral Contraceptives in Polycystic Ovary Syndrome: Risk Benefit Assessment." *Seminars in Reproductive Medicine* 26(1): 111–20.

69

Adenomyosis: Imaging and Treatment

Magued Adel Mikhail, Candice P. Holliday, and Botros Rizk

Introduction

Adenomyosis is the presence of ectopic endometrial glands and stroma in the myometrium with adjacent myometrial hyperplasia and hypertrophy. Adenomyosis presents as pelvic pain, dysmenorrhea (10%–30%), menorrhagia (40%–50%), metrorrhagia (10%–12%), abnormal uterine bleeding, and dyspareunia. Adenomyosis is usually underdiagnosed.

Imaging

- Transvaginal ultrasonography (TVUS): TVUS has the sensitivity and specificity of 57% to 97.5% respectively for the diagnosis of adenomyosis. The signs of adenomyosis on TVUS include asymmetry of the myometrial thickness, parallel shadowing, linear striations (sun rays appearance), myometrial cysts, hyperechoic islands, and irregular endometrial-myometrial junction.
- Three-dimensional transvaginal ultrasonography (3D TVUS): The coronal section of the uterus of the 3D TVUS permits accurate evaluation and measurement of the endomyometrial junctional zone.
- Magnetic resonance imaging (MRI): MRI is an accurate, non-invasive tool. Its sensitivity and specificity is the same as TVUS or a little higher, because of its capacity to detect the low-intensity lesions.

Treatment of Adenomyosis

- Treatment options depend on the patient's age, symptoms, and the desire for future fertility.
- Treatment can be medical, surgical or combined.

Medical Management

- The medical management may include: prostaglandin synthetase inhibitors, oral contraceptive pills, progestogens, danazol, and gonadotropin-releasing hormone (GnRH) agonist.
- Oral progestogens can be used to treat the symptoms of adenomyosis, mainly menometrorrhagia and may cause endometrial atrophy.
- The levonorgestrel intrauterine system (LNG-IUS) induces atrophy of the endometrial glands and stromal decidualization to reduce the menstrual blood loss markedly. LNG-IUS provides successful control of menorrhagia and dysmenorrhea when it is used as 20 mcg/day.
- Danazol-loaded IUD contains 300–400 mg of danazol, has a large volume and requires cervical dilation prior to its insertion.
- GnRH agonist forms create a hypoestrogenic environment, resulting in a decrease in the size of the uterus and improvement of the symptoms without change in the infertility. It cannot be used for more than 6 months because of its side effect profile or prior to laparoscopic excision of adenomyosis to reduce the bleeding as it may make differentiation from normal tissue difficult.
- Aromatase inhibitors can be used based on the presence of the aromatase P450 enzyme in the endometrium of endometriosis, leiomyoma, and adenomyosis. The enzyme has the capability to covert C19 androgens to C18 estrogen. More studies are needed to evaluate its efficacy and suitability.

Surgical Management

- Conservative surgical procedures include endomyometrial ablation, laparoscopic myometrial electrocoagulation or excision. These procedures have been shown to be effective in more than 50% of patients keen on fertility preservation.
- Hysteroscopy has the ability to diagnose the adenomyosis foci and treat them by ablation or excision of the lesions.
- Endomyometrial ablation is limited to the endomyometrial junction and has been shown to control the symptoms in 55% of patients for at least 2 years.

Endometrial ablation is likely to fail if the adenomyosis invasion is more than 2.5 mm.

- Laparoscopic myometrial electrocoagulation has the capability to shrink adenomyosis lesions. However, complete removal of the lesions may not be accomplished. The risk of uterine rupture increases afterwards and that is why sterilization is always offered. Bleeding is not common during the procedure and can be controlled by vasoconstricting agents; however, reports are still needed for the postoperative infection or bleeding.

- Excision of localized adenomyosis is an operation that is similar to myomectomy and can be performed either abdominally, laparoscopically, or by robotic assisted laparoscopy. It is usually reserved for younger patients who have the symptoms of adenomyosis, but have not completed their fertility yet.

- If a surgical procedure is not suitable for a patient, there are some radiological procedures that can be tried and that include: uterine artery embolization (UAE) and MRI guided ultrasound ablation.

- UAE is considered to be a minimally invasive and safe procedure for conservative management. UAE is effective on a long-term basis in the conservative management of adenomyosis and is recommended by some authors as the primary conservative method, but it has a 40% recurrence risk and failure rate and the possible need for hysterectomy.

- MRI guided ultrasound thermal ablation of the affected area can be done in an outpatient setting under local conscious sedation.

- Hysterectomy is the definitive surgery for the diagnosis and treatment of adenomyosis once fertility is no longer desired. It can be performed either abdominally, vaginally, laparoscopically, or by robotic assisted laparoscopy.

Combined Treatment

The combination of surgical and medical managements might provide promising results as the medical management has a temporary effect and the conservative surgical managements have 50% effectiveness.

BIBLIOGRAPHY

Bratby, M.J. and W.J. Walker. 2009. "Uterine Artery Embolisation for Symptomatic Adenomyosis—Mid-Term Results." *European Journal of Radiology* 70(1): 128–32.

Farquhar, C. and I. Brosens. 2006. "Medical and Surgical Management of Adenomyosis." *Best Practice & Research in Clinical Obstetrics & Gynecology* 20(4): 603–16.

Kepkep, K., Y.A. Tuncay, G. Göynümer, and E. Tutal. 2007. "Transvaginal Sonography in the Diagnosis of Adenomyosis: Which Findings Are Most Accurate?" *Ultrasound in Obstetrics & Gynecology* 30(3): 341–5.

Mehasseb, M.K., S.C. Bell, J.H. Pringle, and M.A. Habiba. 2010. "Uterine Adenomyosis is Associated with Ultrastructural Features of Altered Contractility in the Inner Myometrium." *Fertility and Sterility* 93(7): 2130–6.

Meredith, S.M., L. Sanchez-Ramos, and A.M. Kaunitz. 2009. "Diagnostic Accuracy of Transvaginal Sonography for the Diagnosis of Adenomyosis: Systematic Review and Metaanalysis." *American Journal of Obstetrics and Gynecology* 201(1): 107-e1.

Wang, P.H., W.H. Su, B.C. Sheu, and W.M. Liu. 2009. "Adenomyosis and Its Variance: Adenomyoma and Female Fertility." *Taiwanese Journal of Obstetrics and Gynecology* 48(3): 232–8.

70

Ectopic Pregnancy: Evaluation and Management

James M. Shwayder

Symptoms

Presenting symptoms of patients with potential ectopic pregnancy include abnormal bleeding, abdominal or pelvic pain, and often a light or late menses.

Laboratory Testing

- Initial laboratory includes a urine pregnancy test (UCG).
- If the UCG is positive, samples will be drawn, but not sent, for a complete blood count (CBC), blood type and screen, and a quantitative serum hCG. These studies will be sent pending the results of the transvaginal ultrasound (TVS).

See further in Table 70.1.

Imaging of Singleton Pregnancies

- Definitive diagnosis.
  - The initial evaluation of such patients is a TVS. A TVS is obtained prior to a quantitative hCG as a definitive diagnosis, such as a definite intrauterine pregnancy (IUP) or definite ectopic (EP), may be made with this study.[1]
  - The findings consistent with a definite diagnosis include an embryo, with or without cardiac activity, or a gestational sac with a yolk sac either in an IUP or EP location.[1]
  - Waiting for a quantitative hCG and deferring ultrasound until a level of 1000 mIU/mL is reached has two issues: (1) up to 50% of ruptured ectopic pregnancies have an hCG <1000 mIU/mL,[2,3] and (2) the threshold level with modern equipment for identifying an IUP is 390 mIU/mL.[4]
- Determining fetal viability.
  - If the diagnosis of a *definite IUP* is made, the issue is then the viability of the pregnancy.

- New guidelines have deemed that the lack of embryonic cardiac activity, i.e., a missed abortion, cannot be definitively made until the crown rump length (CRL) is ≥7 mm.[5]
- There is little value in obtaining serial quantitative hCG levels once an IUP is identified.
- The status of the pregnancy is best determined by serial TVS.
- In general, the CRL increases 1 mm per day. Some clinicians defer follow-up for 1 week to allow a definitive change in pregnancy development. In those cases with vaginal bleeding, a type and screen is sent to determine if RhoGAM is indicated.
- Ectopic pregnancy management.
  - If the diagnosis of a *definite EP* is made, then a quantitative hCG, CBC, and type and screen are sent for processing.
  - If hemodynamically unstable, then surgical management is urgently pursued.
  - If the patient is hemodynamically stable, then the choice of medical or surgical treatment is dictated by the level of the hCG or the patient's past history.
  - Failure of medical treatment, e.g., methotrexate, is more common if the initial hCG >5000 mIU/mL (13% failure) or if cardiac activity is present (11% failure).
  - Patients with a prior tubal ligation or prior treatment of an EP in the same tube with methotrexate are better candidates for initial surgical management, regardless of the hCG level.
- Lack of a definitive diagnosis by ultrasound.
  - The challenge arises when a definitive diagnosis is not possible.
  - A pregnancy is more likely to be intrauterine if there is sac-like structure within the endometrial cavity, particularly if eccentrically implanted. In fact, the presence of a smooth-walled anechoic intrauterine cystic structure

without an adnexal mass has greater than a 99% chance of being an IUP.[6]

- Conversely, a pregnancy is more likely an ectopic if there is a lack of intrauterine fluid (83% of EP have no intrauterine fluid)[6] and if an adnexal mass is present, a finding with 87% of EP.[6]
- The probability of an ectopic pregnancy is dependent on the adnexal findings.[7] A hyperechoic ring with a sonolucent center, a "tubal ring," has a 95% likelihood of being an EP, whereas any mass separate from the ovary, other than a simple cyst, has a 92% likelihood of being an EP.

- Pregnancy of unknown location (PUL).
  - Pregnancies without identified sac-like structures or adnexal masses are deemed pregnancies of unknown location (PUL).[1]
  - In these instances, serial quantitative hCG levels are crucial for diagnosis.
  - An initial hCG level is followed by a repeat level in 48 hours.

- Normal intrauterine pregnancies rise a median of 2.24 times over 48 hours (range 1.53–3.28).[8]
- The lack of a normal rise should enhance one's suspicion of an EP, or at least an abnormal pregnancy. Some caution is warranted as up to 15% of normal pregnancies have an abnormal rise in hCG.
- TVS findings are then correlated with the hCG levels.
- A thin endometrium is concerning as an endometrial thickness ≤8 mm is associated with an abnormal pregnancy, whether extra- or intrauterine, in 97% of cases.[9]
- The discriminatory level is that level above which all single intrauterine pregnancies should be identified. Recent studies have established a discriminatory level = 3510 mIU/mL.[4]
- Of note, patients with stable or decreasing hCG levels may be appropriate for expectant management as spontaneous resolution occurs in 88% of such patients when the initial hCG is <200 mIU/mL, and up to 25% of those with an initial hCG >2000 mIU/mL.[10]

TABLE 70.1

Sequence of Testing for Ectopic Pregnancy

Laboratory Testing
1. UCG. If positive, proceed with imaging
2. Samples drawn but not sent initially:
   a. CBC
   b. Type and screen
   c. Quantitative hCG

Imaging
1. Transvaginal ultrasound/sonogram (TVS) initially[1]

a. Definite intrauterine pregnancy (IUP)	
i. Embryo with or without cardiac activity	
ii. Intrauterine gestational sac with yolk sac	
b. Possible intrauterine pregnancy: Probability of an IUP	
i. Intrauterine cystic structure without an adnexal mass[2]	>99%
ii. Thickened endometrium	N.A.
c. Definite ectopic pregnancy (EP)[7]	
i. Embryo with or without cardiac activity in the adnexa	
ii. Gestational sac with yolk sac in the adnexa	
d. Possible ectopic pregnancy[7]: Probability of an EP	
i. Hyperechoic ring with a sonolucent center ("Tubal ring")	95%
ii. Any mass separate from the ovary other than a simple cyst	92%
iii. Thin endometrium when hCG is below the discriminatory level[9]	
e. Pregnancy of unknown location	
i. Lack of definitive or early sac-like structures or adnexal masses	

Follow-up Testing
1. Quantitative hCG
   a. Repeat in 48 hours
   b. Expect rise of 2.24 times (Range 1.53–3.28)[8]
2. Repeat ultrasound (TVS)
   a. Threshold for identifying an IUP = 390 mIU/mL[4]
   b. Discriminatory level = 3510 mIU/mL[4]

Complications

- Multiple gestations, whether intrauterine or extrauterine, do not have established hCG curves or discriminatory levels.
- Thus particular caution must be exercised when evaluating patients who have undergone assisted reproduction, due to their greater risk of multiple gestations.

REFERENCES

1. K. Barnhart, N.M. van Mello, T. Bourne, et al., "Pregnancy of Unknown Location: A Consensus Statement of Nomenclature, Definitions, and Outcome," *Fertility and Sterility* 95 (2011): 857–66.
2. M.C. Frates, P.M. Doubilet, H.E. Peters, and C.B. Benson, "Adnexal Sonographic Findings in Ectopic Pregnancy and Their Correlation With Tubal Rupture and Human Chorionic Gonadotropin Levels," *Journal of Ultrasound in Medicine* 33 (2014): 697–703.
3. D. Saxon, T. Falcone, E.J. Mascha, T. Marino, M. Yao, and T. Tulandi, "A Study of Ruptured Tubal Ectopic Pregnancy," *Obstetrics & Gynecology* 90 (1997): 46–9.
4. A. Connolly, D.H. Ryan, A.M. Stuebe, and H.M. Wolfe, "Reevaluation of Discriminatory and Threshold Levels for Serum β-hCG in Early Pregnancy," *Obstetrics & Gynecology* 121 (2013): 65–70.
5. P.M. Doubilet, C.B. Benson, T. Bourne, and M. Blaivas, "Diagnostic Criteria for Nonviable Pregnancy Early in the First Trimester," *New England Journal of Medicine* 15 (2013): 1443–51.
6. C.B. Benson, P.M. Doubilet, H.E. Peters, and M.C. Frates, "Intrauterine Fluid With Ectopic Pregnancy: A Reappraisal," *Journal of Ultrasound in Medicine* 32 (2013): 389–93.
7. D.L. Brown and P.M. Doubilet, "Transvaginal Sonography for Diagnosing Ectopic Pregnancy: Positivity Criteria and Performance Characteristics," *Journal of Ultrasound in Medicine* 13 (1994): 259–66.
8. K. Barnhart, M.D. Sammel, P.F. Rinaudo, L. Zhou, A. Hummel, and W. Guo, "Symptomatic Patients with an Early Viable Intrauterine Pregnancy: HCG Curves Redefined," *Obstetrics & Gynecology* 104 (2004): 50–5.
9. S. Spandorfer and K. Barnhart, "Endometrial Stripe Thickness as a Predictor of Ectopic Pregnancy," *Fertility and Sterility* 66 (1996): 474–7.
10. J. Korhonen, U.H. Stenman, and P. Ylöstalo, "Serum Human Chorionic Gonadotropin Dynamics During Spontaneous Resolution of Ectopic Pregnancy," *Fertility and Sterility* 61 (1994): 632–6.

Index

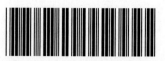